Editing:

Angie Barrett
BSc Hons, BA Hons Education, Midwife, RM, Nurse, RGN

Amanda Burleigh
BSc Hons, Midwife, RM, Nurse, RGN

Dr Patricia Gillen
PhD, M Sc, PGDipE, BSc (Hons), Midwife, RM, Nurse, RN, FHEA

Deborah Hughes BA (Hons) Nurse, SRN, Midwife, RM, MA, DPSM, PGDE

Cover illustration: Copyright © 2023 by Matt Mahurin

Cover and book design: by Suzanne Shepherd

***Disclaimer**

To the best of our knowledge all of the accounts included in this book are of true life events. They were voluntarily submitted to a closed Facebook group in response to the following question: 'Why Do Midwives Leave?' Care has been taken to anonymise all the accounts so that neither the person who submitted the story nor the person/persons/organisations referred to, are identifiable. Therefore, readers are requested not to make assumptions/inferences about the identities of individuals or organisations. The importance and value of the report are not the identities of those within but rather the personal accounts from midwives, student midwives and maternity support workers that provide insight into their experiences of working within maternity services in the UK and Republic of Ireland. The report has been compiled by a group of individuals with the intention of improving maternity services and safety, not with any malicious intent to maternity services, midwifery, or any individual or organisation. It is hoped that these accounts can help to inform the current work undertaken within many maternity care settings to improve the workplace culture and optimise the wellbeing of staff who provide care for women, babies and their families. The term BAME has been used within accounts by individuals, but we acknowledge that updated differing terminology is more acceptable.

Dedication

This report is dedicated to those who have been or who are being traumatised as a result of bullying by their own profession, management and colleagues, including those failed by the systems that are intended to protect and support them such as human resources and workplace unions.

It is also for those who are working or being educated in a system that no longer cares for us and fails to put the women and babies we care for at the centre of our maternity universe.

Respectful and safe care starts with those privileged to give care to women and their families - we are human too and we also deserve to be treated well, cared for, to be respected and to be safe at work.

This report is a compilation and candid record of the collective voices of the #saynotobullyinginmdwifery Facebook group, with thanks to all who bravely shared their experiences.

Foreword

This report will provoke tears and rage. Here midwives and student midwives report their experience of the toxic culture of bullying in NHS maternity services which is so destructive for midwives, mothers and babies. Their words have a rawness which is painful to read. This is not a polished and professional research report. It is cry from the heart by women who simply seek to care for birthing women, presented by midwives who seek to care for their colleagues. This is the experience of so many bullied midwives and student midwives as reported on the #saynotobullyinginmidiwfery Facebook site.

NHS maternity services are in a perilous state with massive staff shortages leading to the exploitation of those midwives who remain and are so often broken not just by the workload but by that last straw: the bullying unevenness of the workload.

Twenty years ago we reported how midwives were leaving midwifery because they could not give the care they wished to give (Ball et al. 2002). Things have got so much worse. Dominated by risk analysis with impossibly long lists of technical tasks which must be done, maternity services have become rigid and fearful, undermining the self-confidence of mothers and midwives. In a service run on a conveyor belt model, so inappropriate for life's most creative work, midwives run to keep up with all the tasks required. Care has been squeezed out in the interests of efficiency (Bunting 2020), yet care is the true heart of midwifery. Despite the rhetoric of woman centred care, the service has become rule driven and rigid: such fertile ground for bullying.

On top of the impossible list of tasks, midwives are exhorted to be "resilient" and "compassionate", whilst no compassion is shown to them. We learn from those around us. Rather that managers caring for midwives and equipping them to care for mothers, students and newly qualified midwives are surrounded by role models of bullying, blame and compliance.

Solving the problem of bullying in midwifery is a major task, not least because of long-standing underfunding of the NHS and changes in wider society and in NHS management. Analysis of the problem and strategies for change are needed, which is not easy in a context where care is so devalued. But the work of the midwives who produced this report and the words of the midwives quoted here, show the depth of commitment to ending bullying in midwifery.

Mavis Kirkham -
Emeritus Professor of Midwifery at Sheffield Hallam University

References

Ball L, Curtis P and Kirkham M (2002)
Why Do Midwives Leave? Royal College of Midwives, London.

Bunting M (2020) Labours of Love. The Crisis of Care. Granta Books, London.

Contents

Foreword 4

Mavis Kirkham -
Emeritus Professor of Midwifery at Sheffield Hallam University.

Glossary and Acronyms 8

Introduction 12

This chapter explains the origins of the #saynotobullyinginmidwifery private Facebook group and why it was set up in 2017. Also, it explains how the group has evolved and the actions and events that have led to this report coming into being.

Amanda Burleigh, Midwife, RM, Nurse, RGN, BSc Hons

Chapter 1 22

Why do Newly Qualified and Student Midwives Leave?

This chapter provides a Thematic Analysis of the accounts of bullying suffered by student midwives and newly qualified midwives in the NHS in the United Kingdom and Republic of Ireland. They were submitted spontaneously to the #saynotobullyinginmidwifery Facebook group.

Jenny Wylam, Midwife, RM, BSc Hons (Midwifery), London Trust and London University

Chapter 2 45

Continuity of Care/Carer

This chapter includes accounts and experiences shared by midwives of issues around the planning and implementation of the Midwifery Continuity of Care/Carer model. It also focuses on midwives accounts of how they feel bullied into changing how and where they work which leads to increased stress, dissatisfaction and burnout.

Becky Millar, BSc Nursing (Adult), BSc Midwifery, MSc Advanced Practice Student

Chapter 3 57

Workload and Safe Care

This chapter includes reports of unsafe and unsustainable workloads, working practices and maternity service culture.

Becky Millar, BSc Nursing (Adult), BSc Midwifery, MSc Advanced Practice Student

Chapter 4 80

Why Midwives Leave?

This chapter includes accounts from many midwives who have been bullied, and as a consequence have left either their job or their profession, at a huge personal, professional and financial cost, to get away from the bully. Some midwives who have been bullied, stay as they feel they have no choice due to family commitments. However, this often has an impact on their health and wellbeing and has consequences for their work, personal life and family.

Dr Patricia Gillen, Nurse, RGN, Midwife, RM, BSc Hons, PG Dip in ED, MSc, PhD, FHEA

Chapter 5 135

The Role of the Unions in the Workplace

This chapter focuses on the important role that unions play in the workplace and the outcomes that may occur when union representation is poor, including the impact on midwives.

Amanda Burleigh, Midwife, RM, Nurse RGN, BSc Hons

Chapter 6 144

Reports and Current Strategies

This chapter identifies the main midwifery unions in the UK and Ireland, reflects on some of the maternity services review reports and how they have evidenced the challenges within current-day maternity services

Jeannine Webster Midwife, RM, BSc in Midwifery, MSc in Health, and Social Care

Conclusion

Karen McEwen, Midwife, RM, BSc Midwifery, MSc Clinical Research Methods 149

Glossary & Acronyms

Not necessrily a complete list but may assist with some medical and midwifery terminology used throughout.

ACAS	Advisory Conciliation and Arbitration Service
Accountability	Responsibility and obligation to explain or justify actions
AL	Annual Leave
Antenatal/AN	Before Birth; during or related to pregnancy
B/Band 5/6/7	Seniority or pay scale
BAME	Black and Minority Ethnicity
BBA	Born Before Arrival (of midwife)
Better Births/BB	The National Maternity Review 2016
BF	Breast feeding
Birthrate+	Staffing and workload acuity tool
BP	Blood Pressure
Bradycardia	Dangerously slow heart rate
Burnout	Physical or emotional exhaustion, involving a sense of reduced accomplishment and loss of personal identity
CIN	Child In Need, safeguarding plan
CLU	Consultant Led Unit
CMW/CM	Community Midwife
CoDH	Council of Deans for Health
Community	Work area outside hospital
CP	Child Protection, safeguarding plan
CQC	Care Quality Commission
CTG/Cardiotocography	A tool used to monitor and assess fetal heartbeat and contractions
DA/DV	Domestic Abuse/violence
Datix	Incident Reporting system

Doula	Trained birth companion
DVA	Domestic Violence and Abuse
ECG	ElectroCardioGraph – heart function monitor
ELCS	Elective Caesarean Section
EMCS	Emergency Caesarean Section
Epidural	Anaesthesia used in labour
FH	Fetal Heart Rate
FTE	Full Time Equivalent
GA	General Anaesthetic
Gaslighting	Covert emotional abuse, making someone question their own reality
Gestational Diabetes	Temporary diabetes diagnosed during pregnancy
GP	General Practitioner
Grievance	Official complaint procedure about unfair treatment
HB	Homebirth
HoM	Head of Midwifery
HR	Human Resources
IM	Independent Midwife
Intrapartum/IP	During labour and birth
Kardex	Documentation chart
LASMO	Local Supervisory Authority Midwifery Officer previous RSL
LME	Lead Midwife for Education
LMNS	Local Maternity and Neonatal System
LW	Labour Ward
MAC	Maternity Assessment Centre
Matron	Very senior midwife manager
MCoC / CoC	Midwifery Continuity of Carer

Methodology	System of research methods
MLU	Midwife Led Unit
MoC	Manager on Call
Morbidity	Disease, condition or symptom
Mortality	Death
MSW	Maternity Support Worker
Multip/Multiparous	Subsequent pregnancy/baby
MVP	Maternity Voices Partnership
MW	Midwife
Neonate/Neonatal	Newborn
NHS	National Health Service
NIPE	Newborn and Infant Physical Examination
NMC	Nursing and Midwifery Council. Professional Regulatory Body of Nurses and Midwives
NNU	Neonatal Unit
NQM	Newly Qualified Midwife
Off-Duty/ERoster	Staff rota
OH	Other Half/Partner
On-Call	Period of time when available to work, usually over and above contracted hours
Partogram	Graph used to plot maternal and fetal wellbeing and progress of labour
PDM	Practice Development Midwife
Postnatal/PN/PP	Period of time after birth
PPE	Personal Protective Equipment
Primip/Primiparous	First pregnancy/baby
Pre-Eclampsia	Serious condition in pregnancy
PTSD	Post Traumatic Stress Disorder
RCM	Royal College of Midwifery. Trade Union and professional organisation

RCN	Royal College of Nursing. Trade Union and professional organisation
Safeguarding	Concerns about welfare which can involve agencies such as Social Services or Mental Health Service
Shoulder Dystocia	Obstetric emergency where the baby's shoulders get stuck inside the mother's pelvis during birth
SLT	Senior Leadership Team
SOM	Supervisor of Midwife. Now Professional Midwifery Advocate Or Clinical Supervisor in Scotland
SOP	Standard Operating Procedure
STM/StMW/SMW	Student Midwife
Supernumerary	Period of time when a new staff member has supervised practice and is not counted within staffing numbers
Syntocinon	Artificial Oxytocin used to induce labour
Tribunal	A forum established to settle dispute or injustice
Trust/The Trust	Organisational unit within the NHS
UCU	University and College Union
Union	Trade Union – an association to protect the rights and interests of workers
Union Rep	Staff member who represents the union within the workplace
Unit	Within hospital
VBAC	Vaginal Birth After Caesarean
VE/Vaginal Examination	Digital examination to assess cervical dilatation
Whistleblowing	Acting in the public interest and reporting information about wrongdoing

Compiled by Becky Millar

Introduction

The #saynotobullyinginmidwifery Facebook group was founded in April 2017.

At that time I had been a clinical midwife for 29 years, and a change agent after I discovered in 2005 that the globally routine and recommended practice of immediate cord clamping was not evidence-based; on the contrary, the evidence showed that early clamping was harmful. I thought changing practice would be easy, as our regulatory body, the Nursing and Midwifery Council (NMC) supports using evidence-based practice in its Code. However, far from easy, the following 13 years of my working life, whilst I was challenging non evidence-based-practice as a clinical midwife, and raising two children as a single mother, were a relentless nightmare. I suffered every aspect of bullying as outlined by the Advisory Conciliation and Arbitration Service (ACAS), which works with employers and employees to help improve workplace culture (ACAS 2022). This bullying led to mental and physical ill-health and culminated, in 2017, in me leaving a profession that I loved (and still do), which has resulted in a very uncertain future for me personally. I was a passionate, dedicated, conscientious and committed midwife and proud to work at the NHS Trust where I trained and did my research (in my own time) for 34 years… I should still be there.

The profound confusion and damage these experiences caused cannot be explored in depth here, but the main injustice was that, despite the fact that I adopted all the recommendations for dealing with bullying, absolutely nothing worked. Diaries, emailing/speaking to management, 'Dignity at Work' representatives, 'Freedom to Speak Out Guardians', writing to the Chief Executive, involving unions, raising a concern, involving HR, completing satisfaction at work questionnaires, occupational health referral (due to work related stress episodes), moving departments, moving hospitals, informing the CQC of bullying within the department … it was all futile. Any NHS employee expects their employer to support their safety in the workplace and to provide adequate opportunities for training and advancement but this didn't happen. Midwives also pay substantial union subscriptions expecting that they will be supported by their chosen union. However I found this support either absent or lacking and this report shows that many members also similarly feel let down when dealing with bullying.

As seems common practice with other "whistle-blowers" (see various accounts in this report), I was investigated and treated as though I was the problem. With my back continuously against the wall, I very reluctantly took early retirement. This was unwise financially but, at that time, emotionally and physically necessary. It had felt very much as though the union, midwifery and corporate management had been complicit in their management of my concern and saw my departure as a problem solved. This theme recurs in many of the accounts the #saynotobullyinginmidwifery Facebook group received.

On reflection, the union and Trust may also have been afraid of what my publicly challenging the harmful practice of immediate cord clamping might bring. I had been awarded local Midwife of the Year in 2012 and National Midwife of the Year in 2015 for my work in promoting evidence-based cord management, yet these awards actually fuelled the bullying and incivility. Just two years after receiving the national award, bullying behaviours led to me leaving NHS midwifery in September 2017. Midwifery just wasn't safe for me.

How did this lead to the group and the report? Throughout all of this time, I knew I wasn't alone. Although the bullying I experienced felt as though it was at an unprecedented level and very visible because of my work on promotion of evidence-based, optimal cord clamping, (and openly witnessed by so many bystanders who did absolutely nothing), I also witnessed other colleagues who also suffered injustices and left the profession too. Great, skilled and knowledgeable, caring midwives who potentially had many more years of service ahead of them, discarded on the professional scrap heap, and who still suffer from these experiences to this day. After feeling let down by unions and management, they left - too battle-weary to fight on, the system stacked against them.

The #Saynotobullyinginmidwifery group was created in April 2017 as a private Facebook support group by myself and antenatal birth educator Dany Griffiths. Within a few weeks we had 1000 members, currently we have over 4000. Over the past six years #Saynotobullyinginmidwifery has been a very active member led group, where members, who include experienced and newly qualified midwives, heads of midwifery, midwifery lecturers, student midwives, maternity support workers and other birth workers receive advice and support and in turn offer other members support and advice. All members are equally important and supported as necessary. Where possible we can buddy members up with other members, which works well with members from minority groups, or students that feel unsupported. We do not profess to offer structured support with regards to employment and legal advice, or medical advice to those who disclose sensitive or mental health issues but we do signpost and support members to access appropriate agencies.

The profession was (and is) haemorrhaging midwives and the situation gets ever worse, year in, year out. The unions highlight that midwives are leaving in droves. However in the evidence presented in this report would strongly suggest that the union itself plays a part in the attrition rate of midwives. Chapters 5 and 6 of this report provide evidence in the form of midwives' experiences and candid views.

"Midwives Matter. Support urgent government investment into maternity services"

In September 2021, Cheryl Samuels (Midwifery Lecturer) started a petition to the Secretary of State for Health and Social Care (UK Government) in order to raise awareness of the crisis in Midwifery. She highlighted reports and surveys, including those by the Royal College of Midwives, which support the dire and unsafe situation that maternity services and midwives find themselves in. She concluded by calling for substantial investment and support for maternity services.

The petition states that "in July 2021 MPs called for urgent action to address staffing short falls in maternity services and an increase in maternity services budget of a minimum of £200-£350 million per year".

Donna Ockenden, in the publication of the Independent Review of Maternity Services into the Shrewsbury and Telford NHS Trust, released in March 2022, also supports and endorses that the amount required to support maternity services is £200-£350 million per year.

To date, this petition has 130,000 signatures of both midwives and service users. Cheryl Samuels updated us to say that the petition was mentioned in parliament by MP Siobhan Baillie in January and Cheryl had a general response from her local MP and also MP Maria Caulfield. Cheryl (accompanied by officials from the Royal College of Midwives and some student midwives) then presented her petition to Downing Street in February 2022. Cheryl has received no responses since the petition was handed in. The petition can be found here:

chng.it/JfCwfKxK

March with Midwives

Alongside the petition, in October 2021, a grassroots movement was started on social media as midwives, doulas, lay-people, families and health care professionals came together to say 'Enough is Enough' and formed the 'March with Midwives' movement. With 23,000 members and growing, this grass-roots movement organised national and local vigils in November 2021, March 2022 and November 2022 in public spaces across towns and cities in the UK.

The demands of this movement are that the government:

Listen

The All Party Parliamentary Group and health ministers concerned with maternity need an urgent consultation with us to undertake a system wide diagnosis to address the immediate crisis.

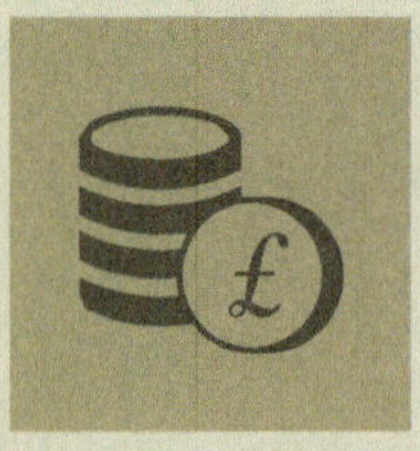

Fund

An immediate, appropriate, restorative pay rise for midwives that reflects the value society places on their vital work. Award recruitment and retention payments for new entrants and existing staff. Provide financial support for student midwives and create posts for all newly qualified midwives.

Enable

Make it possible for self-employed midwives to work, thus putting 250 experienced midwives immediately back into the workforce.

Reduce

Provide £5m of crisis funding to 3rd sector organisations for the provision of breastfeeding support and antenatal education to reduce the pressure on midwifery staff.

Since the formation of the March with Midwives movement we have witnessed a solidarity that has not been felt or witnessed by midwives in a national sense for many years. The collective action of the movement has led, or contributed, to

- Significant pressure on the government to debate the issue of the midwifery crisis in parliament
- A parliamentary debate requested on the issue of the maternity crisis, led by Siobhan Baillie MP
- The formation of an All Party Parliamentary Group for Black Maternal Health, chaired by Bell Ribeiro-Addy MP, calling on the government to set targets to reduce Black maternal mortality
- Public announcement by Jeremy Corbyn MP to call on the UK government to act in response to the demands of midwives
- Significant press and media attention given to the national vigils held in November 2022

Kay King (Movement Director at White Ribbon Alliance UK) and Maddie McMahon (Doula and Breastfeeding counsellor), both members of the March with Midwives steering group, provided the update above and added "We continue to strive towards improved conditions for midwives and health care professionals across the UK as we acknowledge that we are now in a crisis within our maternity services. The collective voices of all who work within the maternity sector, together with parents ensures that we are speaking with one voice as we continue advocating for our demands despite the wider crisis within the National Health System".

In March 2022 the government announced a £127 million funding boost for maternity services across England in order to "help ensure safer and more personalised care for women and their babies". MP Maria Caulfield said, "We want to level up maternity care across the country, ensuring and their children receive the best possible support. Sadly, although the amount is welcome, £127 million is way short of the amount that has been recommended. It is just not enough. (NHS 2022)

www.england.nhs.uk/2022/03/nhs-announces-127m-maternity-boost-for-patients-and-families

As admin of #saynotobullyinginmidwifery, where members regularly reach out to us, and my own experiences, I already knew that the midwifery profession was in dire straits. I believed the group of 4000+ members would be able to help support both these campaigns, so in October 2021 I asked the question on the group "Why do Midwives leave?" Nothing could have prepared me for the tsunami of heart-breaking accounts that I received over the next 2 months. Account after account poured into my inbox from midwives, student midwives, senior midwives, lecturers, ex-midwives, ex-student midwives, heads of midwifery, maternity support workers. Many were happy for their accounts to be published (anonymously) on the Facebook group. Many were happy for their accounts to be passed on but not published on the group page, however, a significant number were terrified of being identified and wished for their accounts to remain completely confidential. The depth of suffering within all of these accounts, without exception, led me to seek advice and I was advised to approach the Chief Midwifery Officer in England, Jacqueline Dunkley-Bent (in post until 12th May 2023). The Facebook Group members were asked and granted permission for us to share a number of these anonymised and confidential accounts with the Chief Midwifery Officer only and we sent her a smaller document containing accounts (approximately 20,000 words). The Chief Midwifery Officer in England was horrified at the accounts that had been shared with her. As a result of this and other associated intelligence about bullying and harrassment, she set up a National Maternity Health and Wellbeing Taskforce which involved maternity care providers, service users and external bodies in an attempt to try to understand and tackle the ingrained culture of bullying, incivilty and disparity in maternity.

It quickly became apparent that these accounts were personal: people were damaged and many had or were having mental health and financial crises due to their experiences, but also due to the lack of resolution in so many of these cases. It seemed that these midwives had not had the chance to voice what had happened to them and to have that voice heard. Simply asking that question gave members the opportunity to voice the distress that they had experienced in a safe space and this resulted in the huge volume of accounts. Each of the messages required a personal response, which often led to dialogue and the promise that the accounts, with consent, would be used to inform and create change. Whilst anonymising all the cases in order to preserve confidentiality, help was then requested. Members of my former Trust who had also experienced bullying and had left the NHS came forward to offer their support and ideas and, over time, the group grew to include a range of colleagues and friends who were keen to help to get the voices of these student midwives, midwives and other workers in midwifery heard.

All the stories were anonymised, put into one document and then each story was placed into subsections.

The chapters are:

Chapter 1: Newly Qualified Midwives and Student Midwives.

Chapter 2: Continuity of Care/Carer.

Chapter 3: Workload and Safe Care.

Chapter 4: Why Midwives leave?

Chapter 5: The Role of the Unions in the Workplace.

Chapter 6: Reports and Current Strategies

There was a section for Solutions, as recommended by the members but it was a group decision that, as this section is so large and complex, it requires special consideration and a volume of its own, which will be evaluated and created separately.

Initially, three members took on responsibility for writing and shaping the chapter which best suited their area of expertise in their own style; one of the chapters, due to its size, was split into two chapters.

Professor Mavis Kirkham an academic who has a wealth of experience studying bullying and incivility, was approached and very kindly agreed to write the foreword to the report.

During discussions, it was agreed that the best format for this document would be a report. Although, we were uncertain about who would be the final audience, we needed to reach an audience comprised of people who would be suitably upset, enraged and powerful enough to be able to facilitate real change. We also knew that we needed to share with the Heads of Midwifery, Heads of Quality Improvement and Education in the devolved countries within the UK and the Republic of Ireland, therefore it was both courteous and prudent that we involve a midwife from each of those countries.

It was a huge ask and members were either approached or volunteered; they were chosen due to their passionate voice in the community. We have a small but very tight team of 10 members. Five of us were also invited to join the Health and Well-being Taskforce and Expert Reference Group which helps keep the Taskforce focused.

Whilst reading through the accounts we realised that there was a common theme of many members being let down by unions, who they described as being complicit/ friends with managers/perpetrators, often the reps were the managers. There seemed to be a lack of willingness to raise grievances or tribunals. The result being more a case of smoothing things over, not really dealing with the bullying situation which left the members' vulnerable and the bullying continuing. Grievances and tribunals were not raised and the union solicitor often rejected cases, which were later found to have been cases that would have had a good outcome for the member. Facebook group members who contacted outside advice and were found out had union support withdrawn. Quite often the result led to the victim leaving the profession completely or retiring earlier than they had intended to their financial detriment, leading to them to seek further employment outside the NHS. This is often seen as a successful solution by managers and unions and the situation regarded as solved. Due to many accounts describing sub-optimal union support, it seemed essential that we included additional chapters about the role of Unions, report and current strategies written by existing members of the team. Members who had left the profession or moved jobs, were not informed they had grounds for employment tribunals, many finding out when it was too late.

Along with the members of the team, a further midwife who has also left the NHS due to bullying and harassment has provided the resources for producing the report.

The #saynotobullyinginmidwifery group members have been updated and consulted regularly during the formation of this report. The report contains the members' accounts and belongs to the members of the #Saynotbullyinginmidwifery group.

Amanda Burleigh, Midwife, RM, Nurse RGN, BSc Hons

References

ACAS/Making working life better for everyone in Britain. Retrieved 30/08/22 from https://www.acas.org.uk Accessed 16th August 2022

www.change.org

Health & Social Care Committee (2021) Workforce Burnout and Resilience in the NHS and Social Care House of Commons

"Midwives Matter. Support urgent government investment into maternity services". Change.org petition, retrieved from https://chng.it/JfCwfKxK 30/08/2022

NHS England. NHS England announces £127 million maternity boost for patients and families. Retrieved from **www.england.nhs.uk/2022/03/nhs-announces-127m-maternity-boost-for-patients-and-families/ 30/08/2022**

Ockenden, D. (2020) *Ockenden Report: Emerging Findings and Recommendations from the Independent Review of Maternity Services at the Shrewsbury and Telford Hospital NHS Trust* Department of Health and Social Care, HM Government

Chapter 1:
Newly Qualified Midwives and Students

"Something is terribly, terribly broken, and if it doesn't get fixed it will break everyone working within the system, like it very nearly broke me."

Thematic Analysis of the Accounts of Bullying suffered by student & newly qualified midwives in the NHS in England submitted spontaneously to the #saynotobullyinginmidwifery Facebook group.

Introduction

There is a problem in NHS midwifery: midwives are frequently suffering from mental and physical health problems, burnout, and leaving the profession in droves (Royal College of Midwives [RCM], 2021). The consequences for antenatal, intrapartum, and postnatal services are potentially very serious: increasing morbidity and mortality for both babies and mothers, as well as a greater likelihood of experiences of trauma for birthing people and for healthcare professionals (RCM, 2021).

The Facebook group #saynotobullyinginmidwifery has been a 'safe space' for midwives all over the UK to share their experiences of bullying, working conditions, and treatment within maternity services. However, 2021 saw an exponential increase in distressing accounts of these experiences being submitted by individuals spontaneously (but with permission to share anonymously) to the group and in response to one another.

Methodology

This thematic analysis includes 87 accounts of bullying within maternity services: 37 from newly qualified midwives (NQMs), and 50 from student midwives (STMs). The groups of individuals that these accounts came from cannot be compared to and/or deemed representative of all STMs and NQMs working in UK and Ireland as it is a self-selecting sample of people who have had negative experiences. However, we know from research by Gillen et al (2009) and Carter et al (2013), and the RCM's investigations and reports on why midwives leave and workforce burn-out (2016 & 2020), that 20-33% of midwives have experienced bullying. As such, the accounts are relevant and important to explore.

Initially, the accounts were taken from the Facebook group and the raw content was saved. Each account was identified as from a STM or NQM and then transferred to the qualitative data analysis software application, NVivo. From here, the identification and coding of trends was undertaken, and themes emerged.

The themes include bullying, unkind, unsupportive, unsafe, and unprofessional behaviour from experienced and senior midwives towards junior staff and learners; NQMs and STMs feeling undervalued and not listened to by management (at all levels); a general resistance (from managers) to facilitate flexible working and enable a healthy work-life balance for staff; and units being run with dangerously low staffing levels.

To keep this report reasonably succinct and easy to read, each theme will be briefly presented with a few relevant quotes to demonstrate the trends. However, there are many quotes from the accounts that should be highlighted. As such, these excerpts are included in a separate section at the end of this chapter.

Results

Despite the difference in status of these groups of individuals, (student v qualified), their stories see the same themes and outcomes emerging consistently.

Experiences of Individuals:

Unsupported, Understaffed and Unsafe

Previous studies (Longworth, 2012, Avis et al, 2013, Randle, 2001, Kirkham, 1999) have proven the importance of student and preceptee midwives feeling adequately supported, in the clinical environment, for them to integrate theoretical knowledge into their practice and become fully competent and safe practitioners. Furthermore, the idea that basic needs must be met before learning and assimilation can occur, is one of the fundamental concepts of Maslow's Hierarchy of Needs (1943) from his Theory of Human Motivation (Weiss & Li, 2020).

As such, it is disappointing that many of the NQMs report feeling unsupported in their new roles as registered midwives. Often, this appears to be the result of poor staffing rather than deliberate behaviour. One NQM stated: *"Lack of support was another key factor - not because the staff don't want to, but they're so busy that they simply can't."* Whilst another describes how *"The postnatal ward was very understaffed and a frightening place to work. Staff did not help or support one another as all were under too much pressure."* Poor staffing has also affected STM experiences too: *"I've had to say no to doing certain things by myself, or have had to get the midwife on multiple occasions before doing things that must be observed. I am often made to feel like I'm being a pain but I know it is the safest thing to do."* Another writes: *"we are often counted in the staff numbers and relied upon."*

However, in some cases, the lack of support does seem to have a malicious intent behind it, and include bullying behaviours: *"Belittling, comments, whispering, and an absolute lack of guidance. Being made fun of if I didn't know anything and nobody showing you what to do "you're in your blues now"."* And, *"She didn't allow me any supernumerary time at all and in fact allocated me more women and babies than all the other midwives."*

Furthermore, some accounts describe episodes in which those midwives, refusing to be supportive, would then appear to enjoy seeing their junior colleagues struggle: *"Beds would begin to block up and I got eye rolls and comments like "work faster!" I couldn't possibly work faster... my shifts were impossible. Time critical tasks fell behind and I was smirked at..."*

STMs had similar experiences too: *"There were never enough midwives for the amount of students in our trust, with some refusing to take students at all and saying openly how they hate us."* Another quote: *"I was frequently penalised, made to feel like an outsider, not accepted within the team and treated differently to other students, including by the student facilitator, and it was apparent to the others in my cohort."*

Whatever the cause, many of the accounts describe bullying behaviours and how the lack of support to NQMs and STMs is enabling or leading to unsafe practice and putting the lives of mothers and babies at risk:

"I'm just waiting for a serious incident to happen. The majority of us NQMs are terrified of going into the unit and making a mistake, because we know the staff are desperate for help but also don't have capacity to properly support us."

"On my first ever clinical shift as a qualified midwife, I was left alone on delivery suite with a woman with numerous risk factors...no support, no break, terrified to leave the woman to escalate to the on-call consultant...ended in a shoulder dystocia and a flat baby who sadly died 12 hours later."

One NQM describes it as *"playing a warped game of Russian Roulette and just praying the tragedy doesn't occur on your shift or with a person you've been caring for after you've gone off shift."*

One of the STMs describes how their *"mentor left me to observe the CTG, telling me I was to use my instincts and let her know if anything seemed iffy. This was a high-risk woman, epidural sited, Syntocinon sited. This was my first shift EVER, about 5 hours into it."* Another wrote: *"Since starting my training I have cared for families and facilitated births alone through severe understaffing. I have pressed call bells that haven't been answered."* Another reports, *"In 2nd year I was left with a labouring woman with a turtling crown, alone and terrified, then got given out to for calling the emergency bell as I should have been able to deal with it on my own".*

Undervalued and Not Listened to

Employee engagement has been found to improve both employee and organisational performance, and higher levels of patient safety (West et al, 2011, West & Dawson, 2012, Dawson, 2018, West & Coia 2019). One of the main ways of engaging staff is through compassionate leadership and listening to the ideas and feedback from employees, involving them in decision making, and valuing their input and work (West & Dawson, 2012, Health & Social Care Committee, 2021). Additionally, research in 1999 found that midwives often felt helpless in a culture of not having their voices heard and where praise is absent. (Kirkham, 1999).

It seems that another common experience among NQMs and STMs is feeling undervalued and being used as a resource with no thought or insight into how such treatment might impact them personally. One NQM described how *"community staff are being forced to work in the acute unit now. They have been rotated too. Some of these midwives have not set foot in the acute unit for 30yrs. They are stressed, scared and feel bullied. The on calls are 'enforced overtime' now. Although non contractual."* Another writes: *"I work in my own time most days. I go above and beyond in my job, but I feel like a number, a payroll number, a resource to be used."* This same NQM states: *"The working environment alone is challenging enough, the lack of time and rest breaks and time to recuperate from shifts is beyond all acceptance, and the level of accountability is beyond all comprehension, and as such I don't understand why people who are meant to be leaders and set by example, are generally the opposite to being 'caring or compassionate' towards their colleagues."*

This Culture is Echoed by the STMs too:

"One particular midwife treated me like a slave and many other students said much the same about her behaviour. I'd be assigned a midwife and work closely with her and STILL be expected to do this other midwife's "studenty jobs"- observations, taking medication to women, answering her buzzers, setting up and disconnecting her CTGs, the list was endless."

Another student describes being chastised for taking time to support women with feeding: *"being told I was taking too much time offering breastfeeding support on a night shift" and that "I wouldn't be able to do that once I'd qualified."*

Not being listened to by managers was another behaviour that makes staff feel undervalued. One NQM writes *"Despite raising these issues, it was always met with "well this is the Cinderella service of midwifery," our legitimate concerns dismissed, despite every ward or area experiencing the same issues."* And another: *"I raised concerns and was told "when you get more experienced, you won't feel so panicky."*

As well as feeling undervalued, not being heard when asking for help puts midwives in situations that are unsafe for themselves and their clients: *"Do I feel unsafe? YES. Do I feel cared for? NO. Do I feel I have rights or even consideration of what's ok for me? Absolutely not. I am a number, a commodity, a prop".* Another NQM writes: *"Despite being assured we were working on 'sufficient staffing levels' I, and many of my more experienced colleagues profoundly disagreed. It wasn't sustainable. We were giving minimal time and inadequate care to our women on both the AN/PN wards despite working flat out with no breaks to rest, and little ability to take 2 minutes to use the toilet.*" These kinds of episodes are corroborated by STMs too: *"We asked our band 7 for help, she said we were managing fine."* Another wrote: *"I was never supported, never listened to."*

Furthermore, all employees in England and Wales have the legal right to apply for 'flexible working', and employers must 'deal with requests in a reasonable manner' and consider the advantages and disadvantages (HM Government, 2022). However, many of the NQMs described how they felt that their requests were not considered fairly, or even led to bullying.

"I was told by one of the matrons that I would have to put in a flexi-working request 'as policy' - and when I did this, the request was rejected 4 weeks after my start date because it was deemed to be 'too rigid' for them to grant."

"I was told that, despite having a severely disabled son who can't just go to anyone (as in childminders etc) because of his extensive needs, I couldn't have 2 set days off per week (the days I struggle with most for childcare) and that I would just have to ask for shift swaps instead."

And shockingly, a further NQM reported: *"they gave me another Team covering an area that was extremely far from my childcare of which I'd arranged with the fact that I was still breastfeeding and I wanted to be in the same area in mind. I told my matron this and she said "Well your child is 1 now so she should be eating food." I wish I was exaggerating but that's what she said. I was given a very busy clinic and was told I could express my milk in the dusty stationery cupboard or the tiny kitchen. There wasn't even anywhere to store my milk. I went on to have mastitis twice and when my child got chicken pox after I was back for only 3 weeks. I took 2 days off and on my return I was taken into a meeting with the new team leader and same matron and told that this cannot happen again and I should have arrangements in place for my child."*

Having seen such situations, some STMs have reconsidered their choice to train: *"I am heartbroken to not qualify but I also have a very demanding home life with a daughter who has a long-term condition. If you can't even get normal breaks, there was never a chance I would be able to care for her and make midwifery work for me too."*

Bullying, Unkind and Unprofessional Behaviour

As well as outright 'nastiness' and belittling behaviour, other types of bullying have emerged in these accounts, including racism, ageism, religious or belief discrimination, collusion and 'gaslighting'("a form of psychological abuse that can cause a person to become anxious and confused and question their own feelings, judgements, and memories." Schechter, 2021). Furthermore, many of the accounts simply refer to the environment as 'toxic':

"I seriously doubt that any sane, healthy, and stable or well person would ever want to remain in such a toxic career and environment" [NQM].

"The atmosphere is toxic, everyone is so demoralised, exhausted and stressed." [NQM].

"The culture there is unbelievable and generally toxic." [STM].

Sadly, experiences of bullying and toxic environments like these are not new in midwifery or the wider NHS, but have been found in previous research (Kirkham 1999, 2000, Gillen 2009, West et al, 2011, Longworth, 2012, West & Dawson, 2012, Carter et al, 2013, Dawson, 2018, West & Coia 2019, Capper 2021).

Belittling and Ageism

One NQM describes how she was *"shouted at and belittled by other midwives in front of other staff and NQM[s]"*. Another writes about how she was spoken to in a patronising and disrespectful way by a senior midwife: *"I was aged over 50, a mother of seven with a senior career in finance behind me. Yet I was treated and spoken to like a naughty child."* A further account of belittling and ageist behaviour included: *"one B7 who talks down to any student or NQM older than herself, ridiculing in the office, talking in code and laughing about other midwives behind their backs and mimicking them, talking about students and being extremely cruel and derogatory."*

There are similar accounts from STMs, with one writing *"one particular midwife seemed to have it in for me from day one, mocking me for my aspirations and belittling me in front of pregnant people and partners."* Another describes how she and her fellow students were abused by the matron on their first day on placement: *"the matron shouted at us, asked us if we were idiots and how we expected to be midwives."*

Furthermore, many of the STM accounts feature their mentors or supervisors threatening to fail their practice assessment documents if they tried to raise concerns about their experiences: *"I, and many of my cohort, experienced bullying by midwives and were treated so badly. We were afraid to speak out because we were constantly threatened by them telling us they were going to fail us." Another student described how her supervisor proudly told another midwife about failing students: "She was rude and abrupt. Then we were doing paper work and her and another midwife were talking about the new NMC supervisor guidance and how they don't approve, then she turned to me and said "I've failed students before and I ain't afraid to fail another..."*

Racism and Religious Discrimination

Again, racism is something experienced by STMs and NQMs alike, with accounts of blatant and more subtle discrimination. One NQM wrote *"I still vividly remember a senior midwife aggressively describing a black woman by a racial slur at handover with over 15 people in the room including a manager who just let it slide, I raised this to the university, but was advised to keep quiet. Ironically, weeks later that midwife won an award for being a great mentor."*

A STM also described how she *"faced and witnessed covert and overt racism as a student midwife during placement. Towards myself, towards other staff, and towards pregnant people and their families FROM maternity staff."* With another STM disclosing *"a few other mentors who made nasty remarks, some to do with my religion too which I always chose to ignore as I feared I would be further bullied or fail placements if I did say anything. (I can't type what they wrote as it's very offensive in my religion)."* And another, *"It was obvious she had issues with my culture and religion. From the start there were a few comments thrown around which I tried to ignore but at some point I came back from lunch and heard a large group of them talking about me and making fun of my writing - I am dyslexic and spelling has never been my strength."*

Collusion and 'Gaslighting'

There is evidence of collusion in some of the examples above, with accounts of overt bullying behaviour witnessed, but overlooked, by other members of the team. There are other accounts from NQMs and STMs of trying to report behaviour, or ask for help from managers, only to find that they were not interested in investigating further, were covering it up or protecting the bullies, or suggesting that it was the victims of the bullying who were simply oversensitive or imagining it.

A NQM wrote: *"I complained formally to management, nothing was ever done to my knowledge, but one of the midwives involved took me aside and told me she knew I "hated her"*. Another: *"When I complained I was told to "toughen up". A STM described how she tried repeatedly to raise concerns and was told "you don't really want to get in to all that" and was advised to take a year out for my mental health. No support, just an 'off you go...'*. Another STM reported being threatened: *"I was told on 2 separate occasions that I shouldn't take it any further or it wouldn't end well for me."* And worryingly, another wrote: *"The system is so corrupt, if you speak out they will do whatever they can to ruin your life. They definitely tried to make an example of me as a warning for other students."*

Additionally, many of the STMs reported that their universities and tutors were no better: *"Our university was aware of the bullying culture and rather than protect us they sided with the bullies, saying that it was a 'personality clash' and that "bullying was too strong a word to use" and "how dare I tarnish respected midwives with that label"*. Another STM wrote: *"The university played the concerns down. They said that this particular person hadn't been brought to their attention before so it was likely a misunderstanding."* These are both examples of 'gaslighting', in which people in powerful positions undermine the lived experiences of bullying. A further student described how she *"cannot approach tutors from the way I have been spoken to, using condescending, threatening and sometimes even racist language."*

Consequences for Individuals

All of the accounts submitted by NQMs and STMs include mention of some negative effect (to a greater or lesser degree) suffered as a consequence of their experiences discussed above. Many have left the profession within a year of qualifying or before completing their training, and many more are planning to. This is supported by the statistics published in the RCM's media statement warning of a 'Midwife Exodus' in 2021. However, more worrying still, every account submitted from both groups includes details of how, from their experience of working in maternity services, their mental health has deteriorated. The following words came up again and again: broken, burn-out, crying, panic attacks, PTSD, and suicide. Sadly, these are all consistent with previous research on psychological distress suffered by midwives (Pezaro et al, 2015).

Health and Wellbeing

Burnt out and Broken

One NQM wrote: *"I left burnt out by bullying and the terror of working on dangerously understaffed wards"*. Another described how NQMs *"are experiencing burnout and are becoming disheartened by the whole midwifery practice, a few I know have or are about to make the jump to Health Visiting, or just leaving the profession altogether."* And one confided: *"I crumbled, I hit the ground running. I couldn't cope any longer with the constant anxiety and panic on shift, the lying awake all night worrying, lack of nutrition. I went off sick and then I left. Now I'm lost and feeling sad."*

A STM wrote: *"I just keep asking myself why am I putting myself and my family through this stress when all that's waiting for me when I qualify is all the same stress but with added responsibility."* Another described how their experience of placement affected her physical and mental health: *"My confidence and mental health suffered so badly that I'd lost over 10lbs in two months where I was barely eating or sleeping properly as I dreaded going into placement."* And another states: *"I have such a heavy heart thinking about how unwell I have ended up because of my training."*

Panic Attacks, Psychological Trauma, and Suicide Attempts

Three of the 37 NQMs who submitted accounts described having panic attacks due to their experiences at work: *"I've never suffered panic attacks but those managers watched me have them, in their office, coming out of the toilets looking tearful, in sluices, and they did nothing to address the seriousness of their actions. Rather the more they saw my sadness the more they went for me."* Another wrote: *"I know I'm not alone in having panic attacks when arriving at work and having to literally force myself to get out of my car."* And: *"Until my final day, less than a year into my NQM post, where I rotate back to labour ward. I have a panic attack in the changing room and know I have to leave."*

This occurrence is increased amongst STMs with 11 of the 50 accounts chronicling their panic attacks. *"My mental health spiralled down and out of control and I had my first panic attack of 7 years whilst in a meeting with my (very unsupportive and patronising) head of midwifery."* Another STM writes: *"I started getting acute chest pains, struggling to breath and feeling dizzy and sick as I was on my way to work, when I got into the office it got worse so I decided to go home, as soon as I was in my car the symptoms started easing and by the time I got home I felt fine. That's when I realised it was an anxiety induced panic attack."* With others still dealing with the legacy of poor mental health: *"I am still getting therapy for the panic attacks I experience."* And: *"There is a definite PTSD lingering in me from my experience as*

I felt anxious just writing it all down." As well as: *"I can't give you all the details as it's just too triggering for me - in fact just reading the messages in the group has been really hard for me and has brought back so many dark memories."*

Many of the NQMs also mention being traumatised by their experiences too: *"I still cannot believe the level of stress and trauma this caused myself, my family and my colleagues, and how it has negatively affected my career overall. I sincerely believe that I suffer PTSD from this experience, which has negatively impacted on my working hours and my ability to be able to spend as much time working."* Another wrote that they: *"Ended up leaving clinical practice as I was so traumatised."*

Furthermore, there were accounts in both groups from individuals who had considered, or attempted suicide. *"It all became too much and I tried to take my own life"* wrote one NQM. While another recalls: *"driving to work in labour ward thinking if I just crash my car maybe I won't need to go."* A STM describes how they *"suffered from constant anxiety and was exhausted. I got so bad I wanted to kill myself."* Another wrote: *"I would return home crying most days and became suicidal from the fear and treatment at this trust."* This STM left during their second year because they were *"repeatedly driving home thinking about crashing my car into a wall."*

Leaving Midwifery

After reading the above, it is no surprise that, of the 37 NQMs who submitted their accounts, 56% (n21) of them have already left the profession (often within months of qualifying), and a further 27% (n10) are seriously considering leaving. Many of the accounts express a sadness at choosing to leave midwifery: *"I loved my midwifery training but only lasted 8 months post qualifying. I thought it was my dream career."* Another writes: *"I was both sad and relieved to leave. I would not return."* And: *"I've wanted to be a midwife my whole life and it fills me with sadness that I lasted less than a year."*

The 10 NQMs who are planning to leave tell similar accounts, with one writing: *"I adore my job, but in all honesty I cannot put it in front of my own mental health. I am completely heartbroken, but there are limits to what you can put yourself through."* Another says: *"it's been pure hell, staffing, workload and bullying has pushed me close to leaving the career I've worked towards all my life."*

As mentioned earlier, many of those who have left describe how they are still suffering from the effects of bullying: *"I handed in my notice. I physically couldn't return due to crippling anxiety and was signed off work. I felt, and still feel like a failure."* And: *"I went off sick and then I left. Now I'm lost and feeling sad"*.

Sadly, again, these decisions and consequences are echoed by the STMs in their accounts too, with 28% (n=14) of those who posted their experiences having left during their training, and another 12% (n=6) on completion. Of the STM accounts, some mention feeling relieved to have left, rather than the sadness cited by the NQMs. One who left before qualification wrote: *"I 100% don't regret leaving, I'm almost certain that even if I did qualify, I would have left within months."* Another states, having read the accounts that others had posted: *"Reading all of these makes me so (selfishly) grateful that I decided to leave my course."*

However, the majority, like many of the NQMs, cite a need to leave in order to protect their mental health. A STM who left during their training writes: *"I have decided not to return, life is too short to suffer for a career."* Another states: *"I eventually came to the difficult decision that I did need to leave for my mental and physical health, because I had started to become unable to care for myself or my children due to the stress."* A further STM wrote: *"I decided to quit for my health and my family. After seeing how unhappy and stressed the midwives are I would never want this job."*

Several the STMs who left the course or decided not to work as midwives upon the completion of their training, described how their view of midwifery changed through being exposed to the bullying and 'toxic' culture in maternity services. One STM who left after finishing the programme describes how they *"dragged myself to the end of 3rd year and finished my degree (still don't know how I managed it) but I knew I DID NOT want to be in the storm of midwifery."* Another current STM wrote how their experience *"has helped me to decide not to be a midwife when I graduate, I'm going to continue and pass my course and do my best to give my best midwifery care as a student despite the challenges."* While one of the STMs who left before qualification said: *"The whole situation changed my entire perspective, from one of excitement and optimism to complete and utter terror and pessimism. I left within 6 months."*

Conclusion

The 87 accounts included in this analysis were stark reading. A number of common themes quickly emerged, and the consistency of these experiences, from across the country, suggests that the culture of bullying student, and newly qualified practitioners, within the midwifery profession is endemic. What's more, it appears that through a lack of acknowledgement and action, those in positions of authority are colluding in, and sometimes leading, this ethos within maternity services.

Several of the accounts describe discrimination of individuals, including those with protected characteristics such as race, age, and religion (HM Government, 2010). Many of these victims are too frightened to speak up in case they experience further bullying. Others who have tried to raise concerns with the Trust or university are 'gaslighted' into thinking that the problem is with themselves, rather than those who are carrying out the bullying.

This discrimination, and bullying is damaging. Not only to the individuals subjected to it, but the midwifery profession, and to maternity services, as a whole. The accounts reflect how this damage results in the uncompassionate care of women and their babies, underpinned by unsafe practice. Many of the student and newly qualified midwives chronicle how the destructive effects that the bullying, demanding and inflexible working conditions, and feeling undervalued and not listened to, manifest in the deterioration of the health and well-being of those suffering it. Resulting in long-term mental trauma, individuals leaving the profession altogether, or in too many cases, the ideation of, or attempt at, suicide. This, in turn, reduces staff numbers and increases the workload of those who remain, who then become victims of burnout and stress themselves. The cycle continues and we see it reflected in the reports of poor Trust performance – with very real, human consequences - such as Ockenden (2022), Morecambe Bay and East Kent (Kirkup, 2022).

However, there is hope. A lot of those who wrote the accounts mentioned that there were some exceptional midwives who supported them. Often enabling and encouraging them to keep striving to provide the best care to women and their families. One STM wrote: *"Some midwives are angels in disguise,"* and another: *"I was welcomed with a very bright good morning. Even just this is enough to change the whole day! I cannot describe what a difference it is to have supportive and nurturing mentors."*

Collating and analysing these accounts is just the beginning: The experiences of a self-selecting sample of participants who posted on a Facebook group dedicated to highlighting bullying in midwifery give a taster of the nature of the problems in maternity services, as perceived by newly qualified and student midwives. However, it would be of great value to undertake further research, selecting and interviewing participants from throughout the maternity services, from all levels of seniority, to further understand the extent of the problem, to explore what works and what doesn't during training of new midwives, and begin to formulate institutional and cultural change to improve the situation for everyone: healthcare professionals and service-users alike.

Hopefully, through bringing these experiences to light, there is a chance for midwifery to recover its true ethos and return to its caring, compassionate, and supportive roots.

Jenny Wylam, Midwife, RM, BSc Hons (Midwifery) London Trust and London University

References

Avis, M., Mallik, M. & Fraser, D. (2013) *"Practising under your own PIN" – A description of the transition experiences of newly qualified midwives* Journal of Nursing Management 21:1061-1071

Carter M., Thompson N., Crampton P., Morrow G., Burford B., Gray C., & Illing, J. (2013) *Workplace Bullying in the UK NHS: a questionnaire and interview study on prevalence, impact and barriers to reporting* British Medical Journal Open 2013; 3:1-12

Dawson, J. (2018) *Links Between NHS Staff Experience and Patient Satisfaction: Analysis of Surveys from 2014-2015* NHS England

Gillen P., Sinclair M., Kernohan W.G., (2009) *Student Midwives' Experience of Bullying* Evidence Based Midwifery 7(2):46-53

Health & Social Care Committee (2021) *Workforce Burnout and Resilience in the NHS and Social Care* House of Commons

HM Government (2010) Equality Act retrieved 07/03/2022 from **www.legislation.gov.uk**

HM Government (2022) Flexible Working Gov.uk retrieved 07/03/2022 from **www.gov.uk/flexible-working**

Kirkham, M. (1999) *The Culture of Midwifery in the National Health Service in England* Journal of Advanced Nursing 30:732-739

Kirkham, M. & Stapleton, H. (2000) *Midwives' Support Needs as Childbirth Changes* Journal of Advanced Nursing 32(2)465-472

Kirkup, W. (2015) *The Report of the Morcambe Bay Investigation* The Stationery Office

Kirkup, W. (2022) *Reading the Signals: Maternity and Neonatal Services atin East Kent - The Report of an Independent Investigation* Department of Health and Social Care, HM Government

Longworth, M. (2012) *An Exploration of the Perceived Factors that affect the*

Learning and Transfer of Skills taught to Student Midwives Midwifery 29:831-837
Maslow, A. (1943) *A Theory of Human Motivation* Psychological Review 50:37-396

Ockenden, D. (2020) *Ockenden Report: Emerging Findings and Recommendations from the Independent Review of Maternity Services at the Shrewsbury and Telford Hospital NHS Trust* Department of Health and Social Care, HM Government

Pezaro, S., Turner, A., Clyne, W., & Gerada, C. (2015) *"Midwives Overboard!" Inside their hearts are breaking their makeup may be flaking but their smile still stays on* Women and Birth 29(3)e59-e66

Randle, J. (2001) *The Effect of a 3-year Pre-registration Training Course on Students' Self-esteem* Journal of Clinical Nursing 10:293-300

Royal College of Midwives (2016) *Why Midwives leave- revisited* Royal College of Midwives

Royal College of Midwives (2020) *The Royal College of Midwives' response to Workforce burnout and resilience in the NHS and social care* Royal College of Midwives

Royal College of Midwives (2021) RCM Warns of Midwife Exodus as Maternity Crisis Grows RCM Website retrieved 09/03/21 from **www.rcm.org.uk**

Schecter, N. (2021) Gaslighting: the signs you are being emotionally abused Netdoctor retrieved 07/03/2022 from **www.netdoctor.co.uk**

Weiss, P. & Li, S. (2020) *Leading Change to Address the Needs and Wellbeing of Trainees during the Covid-19 Pandemic* Academic Pediatrics 20(6):735-741

West, M., Dawson, J., Admasachew, L. & Topakas, A, (2011) *NHS Staff Management and Health Service Quality: Results from NHS Staff Survey and Related Data* Department of Health & Social Care

West, M. & Dawson, J. (2012) *Employee Engagement and NHS Performance* Kings Fund

West, M. & Coia, D. (2019) *Caring for Doctors, Caring for Patients* GMC

Highlighted Quotes from NQM Accounts

Excerpts of some of these quotes have been used in the main body of this work, and are also included in the following longer quotes.

"One band 7 in particular has taken a dislike to me and speaks to me appallingly in front of everyone - so much so that HCAs and other midwives have checked in on me after witnessing the way she is with me. She didn't allow me any supernumerary time at all and in fact allocated me more women and babies than all the other midwives. When I ask questions she scoffs, ignores me or has even given me the wrong answer (witnessed by another NQM who told me she had asked the same question the day before and was given a completely different and more reasonable answer)."

"One B7 who talks down to any student or NQM older than herself, ridiculing in the office, talking in code and laughing about other midwives behind their backs and mimicking them, talking about students and being extremely cruel and derogatory."

"I was told I was 'too polite' for the 'posh' way I spoke on the phone/saying please and thank you too much! Midwife colleagues criticised me for 'still' breastfeeding my child at two years!."

"I was pregnant again towards the end of my time there and had two shifts off sick. Both times I had to present myself on a day off, driving an hour each way to do so, to explain my sickness absence in a formal meeting with an HR representative - for just 2 shifts missed in 1.5 years!."

"There is an unnerving level of hostility, and it's very difficult to be an effective advocate in that type of culture, you either comply or you don't fit in."

"At almost every turn the claws of seniority are about with their constant unnecessary controlling and coercive behaviours towards midwives and nurses."

"I left only 12 months after qualifying, mainly because of shift patterns/family life balance & not wanting my life to be dominated by on calls etc in the community because of COC. I was told that despite having a severely disabled son who can't just go to anyone (as in childminders etc) because of his extensive needs that I couldn't have 2 set days off per week (the days I struggle with most for childcare) because my request was too 'rigid' and that I would just have to ask for shift swaps instead."

"The same midwives have been rude, bullied other staff, and created a toxic work environment. I complained formally to management, nothing was ever done to my knowledge, but one of the midwives involved took me aside and told me she knew I "hated her". It was so intimidating. If I was moved to work in the same area as her, I know I would have to leave my job."

"As a midwife, I see the huge stress caused by compulsory rotation. Some midwives are forced out into the community, others forced to rotate within the hospital environment to areas they really don't enjoy working. Everyone has their own specialist skills and likes and dislikes, and feel better supported in one area or another. Midwives go off with stress for the duration of their rotation, cry every shift, or leave the job altogether. It's a crisis, and management don't seem to care. On top of this we are short staffed constantly, incredibly busy, and feel huge pressure every shift."

"On my first ever qualified shift I called an emergency for a baby that was born after an elective needing resus. I was alone in theatre, absolutely bricking it, but the baby was breathing by the time paeds arrived. When I got back into labour ward, the band 7 didn't ask how I was, just shook her head and said "was that really necessary?."

"My story was over before it started...still very painful. I'm happy now in school nursing but will always feel robbed of my mental health at that time & my career that I waited 15 years to achieve. Gone in 1 year as NQM."

"It's been pure hell, staffing, workload and bullying has pushed me close to leaving the career I've worked towards all my life."

"The feeling that you're playing a warped game of Russian Roulette and just praying the tragedy doesn't occur on your shift or with a person you've been caring for after you've gone off shift. Genuinely terrified as a CTG shows a fetus in trouble but knowing both theatres are full and the doctors are in there and nobody answers your bell as there is nobody free as even the Labour Ward Coordinator has a birthing person. There's so many women and no midwives! We're on divert pretty much weekly, but so is everywhere else, so they have to come but there's no room and no midwives. Babies are being born in triage (only one midwife in there now most of the time), on the ward - hell, we even had a forceps on our ward! There'll be 2 midwives to care for 25 mixed AN and PN women and their babies - one night,

4 months qualified, I had to be in charge as I was the most experienced midwife and we were bed blocked on the ward with delivery suite full. Its utter hell."

"Please, please don't say anything that could identify me, my life is hard enough without that. But the midwives are suffering and worst, the women are suffering and so are their babies."

"The atmosphere is toxic, everyone is so demoralised, exhausted and stressed. My friends are leaving the profession in their droves and to be honest I don't know how much longer I can go on and after working so hard to get her I'm so sad."

"I voiced my concerns clearly fairly early on when I realised the transition was going to be challenging, but my new managers never paid any attention. After just a few weeks I was broken - absolutely terrified of going into work. I felt like every shift I was going to make a terrible mistake."

"I've never felt such dread before a shift than a midwifery shift. Although the culture in nursing is shite too, the midwifery dread was on another level. I lasted a year."

"Since qualifying I have felt like I made a mistake entering the profession at all. At almost every turn the claws of seniority are about with their constant unnecessary controlling and coercive behaviours towards midwives and nurses."

"There's just me (newly qualified) and another midwife caring for a full ward of over 20 high risk women (as usual). The other midwife is ill and may have to go home (I panic at the thought of being left in this situation alone)."

"It was my lifelong dream. It became my nightmare."

"I remember coming home one night and hyperventilating into a pillow sobbing."

"On my first NQ shift I was left alone on a night shift in an area I'd never worked and so it continued. Belittling, comments, whispering, and an absolute lack of guidance. Being made fun of if I didn't know anything and nobody showing you what to do "you're in your blues now". I think I could easily get a diagnosis of PTSD, I feel sweaty just writing this. I was generally unsafe all the time risking my [NMC] PIN, my mental health and the care of the women I looked after."

"There is an unnerving level of hostility, and it's very difficult to be an effective advocate in that type of culture, you either comply or you don't fit in."

"I left burnt out by bullying and the terror of working on dangerously understaffed wards. I felt unsupported by management and frequently blamed and accused for small errors. The postnatal ward was very understaffed and a frightening place to work. Staff did not help or support one another as all were under too much pressure. Everyone was just trying to survive. I cried frequently and became afraid to go to work. I loved supporting women, but the toll on my mental and physical health was too high. I was both sad and relieved to leave. I would not return."

"I seriously doubt that any sane and healthy stable or well person would ever want to remain in such a toxic career and environment. The feminist in me would support every midwife to leave the profession and find a career that at the very least isn't abusive, draining and toxic."

"I began to suffer with workplace stress which just got worse and worse and eventually turned into severe anxiety and depression. In August this year it all became too much and I tried to take my own life. The response from work has been really disheartening- lots of emphasis on how 'ill' I am and no acknowledgement of the fact that it is work alone that has made me so ill."

"Every shift in the unit is dangerously short staffed, often more than 60% short of midwives. 1-1 care in labour is a thing of the past, often staff are trying to look after 2 in labour and a postnatal or high dependency care at the same time. Second and third year students are left to run postnatal bays and manage labourers with 'distant supervision'. Staff are dropping like flies to stress, either short or long term sick, and many have left. It's frightening, and upsetting, and stressful. I discovered labour ward is protecting yourself over caring for women and their families. This is wrong on every level."

"There are so many situations I have found myself in at work that have reduced me to tears. I became so physically and emotionally unwell, and ended up being off for almost 6 weeks - I really didn't want to go back."

"On my first ever clinical shift as a qualified midwife, I was left alone on delivery suite with a woman with numerous risk factors...no support, no break, terrified to leave the woman to escalate to the on-call consultant...ended in a shoulder dystocia and a flat baby who sadly died 12 hours later. I honestly thought I would be sent to jail for negligence and /or be struck off the register. Didn't help when I was pulled into the matron's office 5 days later to be told 'let's go through the CTG together to see if you missed anything'! Ended up leaving clinical practice as I was so traumatised."

Highlighted Quotes from STMs

Excerpts of some of these quotes have been used in the main body of this work, and are also included in the following longer quotes.

"I was frequently penalised, made to feel like an outsider, not accepted within the team and treated differently to other students including by the student facilitator and it was apparent to the others in my cohort."

"I and many of my cohort experienced bullying by midwives and were treated so badly. We were afraid to speak out because we were constantly threatened by them telling us they were going to fail us."

"Undermining us in front of staff and women, criticising our knowledge and skills, chipping away at our confidence every shift."

"Midwives would regularly run down their student publicly, in front of patients, families, other midwives, and other students, which was a horrifyingly humiliating experience, and certainly not conducive to learning."

"There was one occasion where she threw some notes at me. She would talk quite nastily about me behind my back and several times I overheard her."

"If I dared ask questions I'd have a dressing down quite publicly in front of other students, midwives, doctors and families."

"The system is so corrupt, if u [sic] speak out, they will do whatever they can to ruin your life. They definitely tried to make an example of me for a warning for other students."

"She has physically pushed my head when I was observing a perineum and used birth as a power tool telling me if I can or can't get the birth depending on how she felt about me that day."

"I found I was undermined in front of women regarding vaginal examinations, where it was evident the woman felt uncomfortable about how I was being spoken to and made to feel stupid when I asked questions or clarified policies. One midwife wouldn't even acknowledge my presence, not even a hello, glance or eye contact when the shift started when walking past me."

"From day one on my first placement I was subjected to incredulous behaviour from senior midwives whose main aim appeared to be to undermine, bully and break down students."

"I was at the point of having panic attacks in the car before going to start shifts and realised I could not do this for the rest of my life. 13-hour shifts without a break, a bite to eat or sit down. Not to mention the amount of responsibility and extra study that's always required to keep up to date. After my 3 years of training, I was so broken I had to leave. I regret it often as midwifery really was a passion for me."

"My escape from midwifery has been a benefit to my mental and physical health."

"I faced and witnessed covert and overt racism as a student midwife during placement. Towards myself, towards other staff and towards pregnant people/their families FROM maternity staff."

"There is a definite PTSD lingering in me from my experience as I felt anxious just writing it all down."

"My first placement went terrible; I was involved in a near miss with a poorly baby which resulted in my then mentor hating me. I used to absolutely dread coming into placement for her constant glares and she went as far as bragging to other midwives she was after failing me the "expletive" student grass."

"I've been too scared to speak out online about it. I stepped off my degree at the beginning of my third year, my placements led me to be mentally and physically ill; under cardiology and passing out on occasion. This was concluded to be anxiety induced."

"I was belittled and made to feel like dirt on her shoe. Other midwives saw this happening but no one spoke up for me. If I dared ask questions I'd have a dressing down quite publicly in front of other students, midwives, doctors and families. I became very scared to ask anything, I'd either try and figure it out myself or ask someone I felt I could trust. I couldn't face going up to the ward to have documents signed for my placement. University twigged something wasn't right, I went from the bubbly person to the one in tears constantly."

"For some students it's impossible to speak up when they see bullying. They don't want to rock the boat. For others (like myself), it's easier to speak up but what ensues is just soul destroying. I spoke up about how I was treated by another staff member. I was told on 2 separate occasions that I shouldn't take it any further or it wouldn't end well for me."

"I've had to step back this year, with the pandemic the 'learning and teaching' and the bullying in my trust it broke me, I'm 31 with 3 (nearly 4 now) children with a customer based, hard-nosed, managerial background for 7+ years I could look after my own, never had my soul destroyed and my intelligence in so much doubt in all my years."

"I get given another mw who bullies women telling them the baby will die if they don't do as they are told. I quit. My Uni tells me I'm doing the right thing. Thanks for the support!!! I was never supported, never listened to."

"I whistle blew on unsafe practice, doing things without consent from women, not being sterile for procedures such as putting in a catheter or VE's, endless bullying, the toxic culture within the maternity unit, transphobia, racism against patients and staff the list goes on. Now I realize I was very silly to believe I would be protected with my union for students and midwives and the trusts own whistle blowing policies. One midwife found out about my whistleblowing by confidentiality being broken and decided to say I was unsafe."

"A few other mentors who made nasty remarks, some to do with my religion too which I always chose to ignore as I feared I would be further bullied or fail placements if I did say anything."

"I still struggle to understand how the trust where I was bullied so badly gets away with it and I keep hearing of more and more midwives who are being bullied there."

"It still bewilders me now how there are so many midwives who treat students and other staff members with such an uncaring and unsupportive manner when we give so much care and empathy to the women we look after. I still feel these experiences affect me a lot."

"I then received an email back from my LME gaslighting me and suggesting that essentially because I had dared to question the process, I must be mentally unwell."

"The hierarchy in these organisations is toxic, and for this reason I am not even sure that when I qualify, I will even want to be a midwife. Our local RCM rep is one of the most horrific bullies I've ever encountered in my life, so it's not even like you can go to her for support."

"I entered uni as a confident happy 50 year old and ended my degree totally broken. I can't give you all the details as it's just too triggering for me - in fact just reading the messages in the group has been really hard for me and has brought back so many dark memories."

"Emotionally as a person I will never be the same again after what I've been through and seen with bullying."

"I literally even started to doubt myself as a person. Am I deluded, am I an awful person, am I truly one way with some people and the opposite with others. I realised I had become withdrawn and I had lost myself in that toxic environment, because they had beaten all the happy out of me."

"I feel it is seen as the norm that being treated badly by the midwives is part of being a student midwife experience. Midwives would joke and ask how many are left on our cohort. How many have left because they weren't cut out for this or mentally strong enough, and if we need to have thick skin to work with the midwives. My family and husband have begged me not to go back as the bullying affected my mental health a lot, triggering panic attacks, low self-esteem and anxiety."

"I just keep asking myself why am I putting myself and my family through this stress when all that's waiting for me when I qualify is all the same stress but with added responsibility. Coming into it I knew NHS staffing was an issue but never in my wildest dreams did I imagine it to be this bad."

"I suffered from constant anxiety and was exhausted. I got so bad I wanted to kill myself. Students and midwives are suffering, it won't be long till someone takes their life."

"I was bullied as a student and ended up on multiple medications for depression and anxiety, got berated for having a panic attack."

"Students have reported that they feel like they cannot speak to tutors due to the way they are sometimes treated in class. If no compassion in shown in the classroom, there is no surprise that lack of compassion is reflected in practice as well. To make matters worse, when students have raised concerns with management, students have been made to feel that they have misunderstood and misinterpreted staff behaviour."

"As a young woman who hasn't had children - but wants too - I'm left feeling scared for when my time comes. It is so clear that midwives are burnt out and unable to give pregnant people the safe care they so deserve."

"I am still wondering if I could have saved the baby if I'd been in a position to make sure he was seen earlier. I suppose I'll never know, but did we practice safely? No, we didn't. We couldn't."

Chapter 2:
Continuity of Care/Carer

"I was safe, kind and able always but I was also hungry, thirsty, scared to ask for help, unhappy to give care below a standard I'd have liked to receive it, and unwilling to be part of a system who had stopped questioning, stopped kindness, stopped smiling."

Following serious issues identified in maternity services and high-profile investigations into failures at a number of service providers in England (Kirkup, 2015), the National Maternity Review (NHSE, 2016) was commissioned to address public and professional concerns. "Better Births" centres around nine workstreams and aims to improve the way the NHS provides maternity care to all women. Central to this is the implementation of Midwifery Continuity of Carer (MCoC) which is proven to improve outcomes including reducing premature births, reducing iatrogenic harm through interventions, and increasing choice and satisfaction with the maternity experience. MCoC involves a Named Midwife caring for a manageable caseload of women in a specific geographical area, and providing all midwifery care throughout pregnancy, intrapartum and postnatal. This is a very different way of providing care in most NHS maternity units where the traditional way of care has been to provide antenatal and postnatal care separately to intrapartum care.

To practise as a midwife requires registration with the Nursing and Midwifery Council (NMC) with a commitment to uphold The Code (NMC, 2018), which reinforces the need to deliver safe care 'on the basis of best available evidence' while prioritising people and putting their interests first. In Ireland nurses and midwives are regulated by the Nursing and Midwifery Board of Ireland. (NMBI 022). If employed and practising within a local NHS Trust, or Board in Scotland, or hospital group in the Republic of Ireland, midwives and all health care providers must work within local and national policies and guidelines. In addition to this, MCoC is included in the Clinical Negligence Scheme for Trusts in England (NHS Resolution 2021) and supports the delivery of safer maternity care.

Despite the known improvements in outcomes and the professional requirement to practise effectively, national and local policy demands care is provided in a specific way, and there is a resistance to change from a high percentage of midwives who are unable or unwilling to change the way in which they work and provide MCoC. A survey in 2018 found that just one third of midwives felt they could work in this way (Taylor et al, 2019) and there are reports of increasing levels of stress and burnout amongst staff who work in this model (Dharni et al, 2021). In addition to this, the effects of the COVID-19 pandemic and national shortages of midwifery staffing (Stephenson, 2020) has led to many midwives being at risk of burnout due to increased demand, low morale and unsafe working conditions (Walton, 2021). Furthermore changes in the way they are expected to practise may mean more midwives will leave the profession and exacerbate the staffing crisis. However, the climate post-pandemic may also mean that more are willing to work in a different way that will improve their work/life balance. Midwives recognise that the maternity system has to change, and Better Births and MCoC provides the opportunity and evidence to do so. However, to be effective, any transformation of services to new models must take account of the needs and capabilities of midwives (Turner et al, 2021). In order to implement MCoC on a wide scale across the UK maternity service, we need evidence from midwives themselves to explore their own reasons for engagement, or otherwise.

The following accounts provided by the midwives focus on both MCoC and workload. They were read and categorised under MCoC and workload and five subthemes within MCoC. The quotes are included verbatim with identifying details removed.

The accounts gathered reveal that midwives feel pressurised into working in a way that they are not used to and have not been given the time, skills and preparation to adapt to. While midwives acknowledge that MCoC is supported by the evidence, the demands of the rotas, and the need to work across all areas with no additional upskilling or recognition of where individuals would prefer to work, makes midwives reluctant to accept this change. The new way of working also impacts on their work-life balance and it is necessary that this needs to be considered and then taken into account. While transformation of maternity services is currently necessary, forcing midwives to work in areas outside of their expertise and comfort zone is perceived as bullying by many midwives, leading to increased stress, dissatisfaction, and burnout with subsequent impact on recruitment and retention of midwives.

Is this Continuity of Care or Carer?

The following quotes from midwives relate to the lack of planning and support for the implementation of MCoC and its subsequent impact on the morale and well-being of midwives. The term 'Continuity of Carer' describes consistency in the midwife or clinical team that provides care for a woman and her baby throughout the three phases of her maternity journey: pregnancy, labour and the postnatal period (NHS England 2017).

"This is so sad. Continuity of Carer is midwifery - with woman throughout her birthing journey. The problem is not CoC it's the way in which it has been implemented. Better Births advised that it would not be possible within the current staffing models and that a radical approach was required! This has not happened; they have implemented a new way of working into an old system without adequate resources. As a consequence, midwives are burnt out and demoralized! Done right CoC works for both women and midwives work life balance can be achieved!"

"When Continuity of Care means a team then it often provides less real continuity for the woman or birthing person than the traditional model of community midwifery with one midwife giving all/most of the antenatal and postnatal care."

"I totally understand the challenges for midwives, but this was totally expected. Under fund it, over pressure it, break it, convince people it won't work."

"Fund and staff it properly with midwives who WANT to do the birth cover and for whom it fits with their lives."

"It has been done and it is possible. But it has to be done with a manageable caseload and that was never going to happen. We started looking at this when we were so far away from it... As you say, not even anywhere near continuity in AN in many places, the change was too huge when it was built on an already broken system."

"But that doesn't mean it can't work. It just means that it can't work without being built from the ground up. And I still hope that at some point that might be something that would happen."

"I will add that I disagree only in the sense that I really want to still see it in place because we know it gives the best outcomes whether it's something people ask for or not. BUT I also absolutely recognize that most CoC implementations since BB have been done in ways which are totally unsustainable and will have caused great stress. This was anticipated by us all."

"Having someone who knows the person in labour to trust their intuition makes a huge difference. I just don't know how it's feasible - it would be so good if it was teams of two or three midwives so the person could be attended in labour by one of three."

The following quotes from midwives highlight their belief that MCoC is possible and preferable for some, implemented with careful planning and adequate resources

"I agree mostly except working in a continuity team was the best, most rewarding time in my career. Done properly - 1) midwives have control of their diary- decided for themselves when they do their appointments and which days/ night they are on-call, 2) organize their own workload- no call ins to cover unit staff shortages, manageable caseloads, buddy groups of 2/3, 3) are supported by management and can work autonomously - design their own SOP, implement what they want or need to function, IT systems are functional, supported by MSW's 4) are paid well for on calls and get more annual leave."

"CoC is possible - WHEN DONE RIGHT it can be amazing for everyone, including the Midwives." Fund and staff it properly with midwives who WANT to do the birth cover and for whom it fits with their lives."

"Being able to build up a relationship with my midwife and knowing it would be her (or her partner) assisting me in labour was THE difference between opting in or out of NHS care."

"I think the carer/care point is such an important one to be clear about ... it's very different - and care is much more achievable than carer. One more thing - the NHS simply cannot provide a 'private' continuity model of care the same as IM can - it's just not feasible and essentially the Continuity model is trying to emulate that provided by IM. How can we do that with such a shortage of staff? We just can't and that's adding to the existing pressures."

Staff Don't want to, or Can't, Provide Continuity

Contrary to the accounts above and the evidence that supports MCoC, these midwives share concerns that providing continuity of carer is not feasible for them given their own personal circumstances.

"The problem is, as shown, a lot of us don't want to do CoC. There are not the midwives coming in who do, so by that logic, it is not going to work."

"What hasn't worked is forcing people into a model that they aren't on board with. It is also doomed to fail if people trying to implement it don't understand the model and haven't had any training in how to manage people and change!"

"I'm a rotational midwife, particularly passionate about IP care (of which one day I will apply for a core position), but am currently in the community and see the hardship fellow colleagues face daily. When in the community, I want to fully support women antenatal and postnatally."

"Women's health is becoming more complex, more and more women with severe, significant medical co-morbidities are accessing maternity services and whilst the theory of CoC is wonderful, the reality of having a CoC midwife who comes to LW maybe 2-3 times a month, is not trained or confident with high dependency care and may not have a vast amount of experience with the relevant protocols etc. Surely having core IP staff is vital to care for the women who can't/shouldn't be having the low risk/hypnobirthing/pool deliveries because they need a continuous ECG due to complex cardiac history alongside pulmonary oedema."

Some midwives while understanding the positive aspects of MCoC, highlighted the pressure that newly qualified midwives can feel under, as they lack confidence and are not given adequate preceptorship and ongoing support. It is not as simple as just being upskilled and then expected to "get on with it."

"How is a newly qualified band 5 who spends most of her time in community going to cope with a pre-term diabetic woman on a sliding scale whose CTG (cardiotocograph) becomes pathological."

"When people are pushing CoC and saying it's wonderful and it improves outcomes, I am often thinking about the above sort of scenario and wondering what kind of evidence they're looking at!"

"I agree, but done properly, CoC midwives end up with a vast amount of experience in all areas."

"Jack of all trades, masters of none."

These accounts highlight the lack of recognition of valuing the specialisms and preferences of midwives for their area of practice.

"I ask why should we? Some midwives recoil at the thought of LW, some midwives really don't enjoy the social work side of community, some midwives thrive in a triage setting."

"Surely when a midwife is happy, confident and relaxed in a setting she's most familiar with... and not forced into a box.... Is when the best care is provided."

"Trusts need a balance of both I think. Those who enjoy CoC can do that, and those that don't can work where they choose."

"I just don't know how I'll make it work with the on calls being a single parent. I like knowing I go to work and my shifts are what they are rather than potentially being called in and then having to work the next day etc. I just cannot see how this is family friendly at all."

"The irony is that in order to be more available to people we are caring for, this means less availability to our loved ones."

"Definitely being able to choose where you work and being excellent there, rather than being made to rotate to all areas and being adequate everywhere."

"Just as I'd like to see the same GP each appointment for a medical condition - but don't care who does the surgery (as long as they're skilled and safe.) Have never understood why it's any different!"

Do Women want Continuity?

These accounts are from midwives who have recent experience of maternity services including MCoC. Generally, women who have experience of MCoC like the experience and want to have that experience again (McInnes et al, 2020). However, there are also some women who are less interested in the MCoC but want kind, compassionate and skilled midwife/midwives to care for them. Some midwives reported women telling them antenatal and postnatal continuity is important. There is support for the MCoC models of care (NHS England 2016; Scottish Government 2017).

"Having experienced true continuity wouldn't a million times want to accept anything less."

"As a midwife for vulnerable BAME women etc I have asked what is important to them answer a caring, competent midwife but to know AN and PN midwife. We have around 80% continuity of carer except delivery, if we were to do MCoC it would decrease. I also talked to an independent midwife, same age as me, and she has dropped intrapartum care but still has plenty of women wanting AN/PN continuity."

"As both a midwife, and also as a birthing person - I did not give a tuppeny who cared for me intrapartum - I just wanted someone kind who was comfortable in that area."

"When I was a CMW we worked in small teams - of about 4 midwives to cover each other. It was fab - in the area I worked my clinics would be covered by the other midwife from the GP across the road. My clients only saw me or her - for the whole pregnancy/postnatal period. They would say they didn't care who looked after them in labour as long as they were kind. I'd often pop into labour ward on my way home and catch up with them, staying a while (if I could)."

"I know as a pregnant woman I loved having the same midwife during pregnancy and postnatally but I wouldn't be able to tell you who I had in Labour and before I was a midwife I didn't care who cared for me at that point."

"Whilst our feedback is great, many women verbalize that they just want someone knowledgeable, kind and compassionate who will listen to them during their birth and labour."

"With both of my kids I didn't really care about knowing my midwife for birth, just that they were respectful of my wishes and practicing & confident in the area I birthed in (MLU for first & at home for second) but I wanted to see a familiar face at appts. And I really HATED seeing a different midwife postnatally, the advice is always contradictory!"

"My second baby was born 9 weeks ago, I had excellent AN continuity bar one appt when my MW was on holiday, but it was far more important to me that the midwives who attended my homebirth were kind, knowledgeable and experienced in facilitating homebirth. I won't badmouth her but my MW was not all 3 of those things. Thankfully my birth midwives were excellent. I then felt very letdown PN as I saw a different midwife each time, whose BF advice all contradicted each other, no one seemed to know my MH or medical history, and I was unceremoniously discharged without decent care at all."

"I've joined 2 'due in...' groups for peer support during my pregnancies and the thing people post again and again is not having a named contact, not seeing the same MW more than once - surely we can't just jump to birth continuity until we at least can say we can provide AN continuity?!"

"There is no doubt that knowing your midwife makes a difference but there are very few women I have spoken to or dealt with over the years for whom knowing the person that cared for them in labour was as important as continuity AN and PN. As long as they have some one kind caring and compassionate who will support their wishes I would argue most women would be happy with that."

"There are so many vulnerable ladies on my caseload, who say to me: 'will you be there for me in labour?' And I would love to say yes ... but even if I was working in a CoC team all I could say is 'well there's a 1:8 chance I'll be there'."

"Those women and birthing people who plan a home birth and meet their home birth team, or a few of their community midwives, they expect to be cared for by these midwives who they know and respect and trust."

"Why should there be a break in the system of care during her/their most vulnerable time - giving birth?"

On-Calls and Escalation

Grave concerns were expressed about on-call and escalation with poorly planned and managed systems that impact negatively, primarily on community midwives and which result in excessive hours of work. This affects the community midwives' own caseloads, safe practice, well-being and work life balance.

"We need to get rid of the on-call system for community midwives. No community midwife should work all day and then be on call overnight or in reality pulled to do a 12.5hr shift in the unit. This needs to stop. In fact you shouldn't be working the day of the on call."

"But then that means being on-call on a day off which equally doesn't feel very appealing!"

"Should never be part of escalation. If needing on-call for when Labour ward is busy, needs covering by the unit."

"Our MCoC team were not officially part of escalation but kept getting pulled so it folded."

"Ensure that on calls are protected for home births - not seen as back up for staffing other areas."

"I really struggle with the potential that I MIGHT have to work ... I would have to arrange potential childcare for those 10 days and that stresses me."

Potential solutions

These are potential solutions provided by midwives which are in support and also against MCoC. The following suggestions all came from one midwife which led to an open, full and frank discussion about the issues that she felt needs to be addressed in order

"Discontinue the CoC model ASAP and return to midwives providing continuity of care in the antenatal and postnatal period with core Labour ward staff for the intrapartum period.

Women mostly want the same midwife during their pregnancy and someone who is compassionate, competent and confident to attend the delivery of their babies...the majority don't actually care or expect to know the midwife who attends delivery...if you ask them ALL...not just the select few who access MVPs etc!

Women who are most in need of continuity (families in deprivation, non-English speaking, BAME women and safeguarding families) are the least likely to come forward with their voices and/or attend MVP events/meetings. (Maybe include a portfolio of all maternity staff with a small blurb/video profile about them on the Trust maternity pages so women can visit and visualise and 'meet' the midwives who may be at the delivery).

Midwives should be able to choose which area they enjoy working in (this is soooo important!!) therefore making a happier workforce who are specialists in their chosen area of work (rather than 'Jack of all trades, master of none'!) and being able to provide robust, competent care to women and babies resulting in better outcomes for women and improved work performance.

Ensuring that community and AN/PN ward midwifery is held in the same esteem as Labour ward staff, are valued, funded and staffed appropriately to ensure a gold standard of safe, compassionate care.

Review of time allocated for AN appointments in relation to care pathway demands…i.e. extend current 20 minute slots to 30 mins to allow enough time for AN checks, bloods, swabs, membrane sweeps, risk assessments, discussions of personalised care plans, referrals etc.

Focus on happiness and well-being of staff in the workplace. There is so much evidence to support improved outcomes and work performance when staff feel supported and valued by their employer!

Allocate quality time for students and mentors to enable discussion/training/ paperwork etc which will help to alleviate the negativity experienced by students from midwives."

The above points from one midwife led to further suggestions from other Facebook group members.

"What about a 36-week birth plan discussion with an Intrapartum midwife from their chosen place of birth?"

"The system needs to change, not the work itself. When women don't get into a CoC model here, they are put back to core staff. Within our model, we also have spots that are kept open for women who may not seek AN care until late in pregnancy so as to ensure that it's not just women who are low risk (across all determinants) seeking care from us when at risk women would benefit more."

"Having someone who knows the person in labour to trust their intuition makes a huge difference. I just don't know how it's feasible - it would be so good if it was

teams of two or three midwives so the person could be attended in labour by one of three. It needs to revamp from the ground up not just at a management level."

"The only way I see a true CoC model is if we become like New Zealand, all midwives are freelance contractors and pregnant women shop around for one, and the government pays the bill. You would only get a couple of women every month to ensure you can be there for the birth and pp period. The way things are in the UK right now I really don't see it ever working out."

"The improvement in outcomes that the evidence shows is marvelous, but if you work in a team of 8 - to make sure that women meet all MW during the AN period you're looking at disrupting AN continuity by having all 8 MW take at least one AN contact each, or the client may have a coffee in a room of all 8 MW ... but how is meeting a caregiver once really true CoC? Is it not better to have a highly skilled MW for who IP care is their bread and butter, rather than a CoC MW who may only work on LW a couple of times a month? Also the swapping over of the CoC midwives at the end of their on call periods disrupts IP care more than having a long day/long night MW surely? I am genuinely not convinced about the validity of the improved outcomes when CoC is given in the fragmented models being rolled out by trusts, when achieving good AN & PN continuity (as we did previously) can be disrupted - surely preserving that and being cared for in labour by a confident and skilled practitioner is just as good? And I've seen many MWs burn out working in this model. At our trust CoC is currently paused as it was unsustainable with current staffing levels, and there is not a single MW I have spoken to who has been temporarily moved back to traditional CM/LW/AN/PN roles that wants to go back to their CoC team. It's killing midwives and it's killing the service and when will NHS England take notice that they've given us an unachievable goal inside a poisoned chalice!"

"I really hope they don't discontinue continuity of care, so many midwives want to work this way and are happy doing so! I think the roll out just needs to be paused in places that are struggling, rather than going backwards and taking it all away. It should be a choice for this who do and those who don't."

"Work on the poor culture of bullying. That's the only concern with people choosing their place of work. Rotation is the only way of dealing with cliques forming."

"Community also need to be respected as much as labour ward staff. Community isn't an easy ride or a cop out, it is as important as labour ward. It is where all the

risk assessments are done so those on all the wards know what to expect from the women (mental health history, DVA, fears in childbirth etc. It feels like a hierarchy at times with community dead on the bottom. They are all vital!"

In conclusion, in order to understand why midwives cannot provide a model of care that has known benefits and improved outcomes, we need to understand the midwives' own lived experience of midwifery and their individual beliefs in their midwife role. There are unresolved conflicting needs and demands between the public perception of the professional being, the requirements of the patient, the employer and professional bodies, with her/his own responsibilities and personal life which need to be balanced. Midwives are themselves a part of the society that they serve and their own parenting and other caring responsibilities cannot be ignored. In an ideal world, all Midwives would unquestionably provide the best possible care and choose to be cared for within a MCoC model.

Becky Millar
Nurse, RN, Midwife, RM, BSc Nursing (Adult), BSc Midwifery, MSc Advanced Practice Student

Chapter 3:
Workload & Safe Care

This chapter relates to the excessive workload that seems to be part of the professional reality for these midwives in today's maternity services. Many of the accounts relate to institutional culture and the repercussions of speaking out. The accounts also reflect the changes these midwives have seen over the years ranging from the 'Call the Midwife' type care where the midwife was a respected figure in the community, to a system where regular escalations of safety concerns to senior staff are needed to provide a basic level of care. Many of the accounts provide examples of where midwives have felt care was unsafe but requests for help were ignored, leaving the midwife unsupported and vulnerable, and impacting on safety of women and babies. The common theme of feeling bullied to work additional hours, or provide care when the individual is unsafe to continue pervades the narratives:

"I have been a midwife for 20 years and from my very first day as a student, I have always felt I was with 'my people', a crew who were kind, caring, intelligent, questioning & compassionate. For me this changed about 5 years ago. The introduction of 12.5hr shifts instantly stopped staff crossover resulting in the removal of: opportunity to seek or give support to colleagues, no natural way to decompress with colleagues & no nurturing of junior staff or students. Exhaustion became a regular feeling as breaks could no longer be staffed- if you took a break your client would have limited to no care in your absence, you had no opportunity to safely use the toilet, no time to read emails & be informed of updates, praise, or the upcoming unit plans. This loss of opportunity to learn or feel part of your unit's, looking back at what once was there but looking forwards no longer was. Staff lost their drive & passion. Each shift became a survival mission with compassion, kindness or smiles removed as options. Students weren't allowed to gain the skills they needed because the shift needed them to continually do the tasks they were safely doing - so teaching wrongly become a luxury. Every department & area was pulled from to cover LW every shift, as staff on shift couldn't pull together to cover sickness or uncovered hours for 12.5 hrs as opposed to [previous] 7hrs (when we

had short staff shifts). Staff were forced to work where they could get childcare for, as most childcare providers 99% of the time offer placements 45mins after a shift had started & remove cover 2 hrs before it had finished, even in the hospital on-site nursery so, without family, covering the 12.5hrs remains impossible. For the 1st time in my career, ***the core LW became elitist as the focus to make sure the ward was staffed over the staffing of other areas gave a superiority feeling.*** *When the outcome of a B7 consultation resulted in the only way to keep my B7 was to move from low to high risk care my enthusiasm for my career disappeared.*

Add to this no support from my manager re a different skill set requirement, defending my banding to other B7's and having to challenge their unkindness, the exclusion from their WhatsApp or social catchups made working hard. ***I didn't tell my manager I was being bullied as for a long time; I thought I deserved their treatment. It took an article in a journal for me to realise it was workplace bullying. Once I spoke up nothing changed & there was no 'the doors open'. I remained alone.*** *Add in failing to gain new roles x4 internal interviews and no direction to improve, self-develop or again 'check in' after constant knock-backs, caring for family - I didn't share with my manager my home life as I feared it would prevent me further from gaining a new post and truly believing any disclosure would not remain confidential, so following a family bereavement when the pandemic came and 6 months later, I couldn't carry on coping.*

I asked an on-call manager 'how much is too much', and finally I was heard. I was sent home; I saw my GP & took 3 weeks off. I returned fearful & wobbly and 4 months later finally realised I mattered. I would only ever be a numbered staff member and if I had any self-worth I needed to leave. I left without a good bye party, without any follow up, simply a WhatsApp message from my manager & a nicely written exit letter. I had started my career so promisingly with a first at uni, gaining my B6 within 6 months, and grew my skills through positions in caseload, traditional community, birth centre, LW coordinator, triage lead & PMA ... I left feeling like an unimportant no-one. It has taken 15 months post leaving to get to a point where I know I was never at fault. ***I was safe, kind and able always but I was also hungry, thirsty, scared to ask for help, unhappy to give care below a standard I'd have liked to receive it, and unwilling to be part of a system who had stopped questioning, stopped kindness, stopped smiling.*** *I feel there is no recovery. Quality care is no longer the priority, the aim is enough care alongside extensive & multiple documenting, without self-care, happiness or team wellness."*

"I am a midwifery lecturer and I have been for a long time and I have never seen it this bad. We have senior management teams pushing us to recruit more students knowing that the clinical area is struggling to adequately support and assess students. Clinical staff are on their knees, yet are expected to complete feedback and fulfil assessment requirements. We are now in a situation where staff just ignore emails, so we as university lecturers have to escalate it (otherwise students do not pass their practice assessments) knowing that by doing so, it will further demoralise clinical staff and add to their poor treatment. **I regularly speak to midwives who are tearful, exhausted and completely demotivated** *- I wonder why we are seeing the largest attrition rate I have ever seen in my long academic career eh? We now ask staff to help with the assessment of students by completing reams upon reams of paperwork: most do it in their own time because they care..... but they shouldn't have to. Part of the problem is the leadership: we have CoDH pushing for us to reduce our standards so we can have even more students (did you see the consultation where they supported simulation in place of some practice?) As lecturers, we are certainly not going through what our clinical counterparts are, but these cultural pressures of working us to we drop are pervading us as well. Health studies are no longer the cash cow that universities depended on, as such I have watched with dismay as we are increasingly taking on admin jobs and meeting quality drivers which gives us less time to support students and resolve some of the issues that other members have flagged up in this thread. My colleagues and I regularly work from 7 to 9 daily and have to work weekends too to keep up. Am not trying to compete: clinical staff have it worse but it does mean that we fail our developing future midwives from the offset. I genuinely think that some of this is due to NMC leadership - how can midwifery call itself a profession when we do not self-govern? The Council do not have any midwives just advisors (there is not a role for nursing advisors on the Council), so we do not have anyone to lobby for us."*

"I am no longer a clinical midwife and this is some of my story - I have redacted a lot of detail as I don't want to be identified. I have just highlighted the occasions where my needs were not met and/or I felt my working conditions were unsafe. As a student midwife I reluctantly returned from maternity leave breastfeeding 10 months after the birth. I considered not returning as I already had realised midwifery would have to come before the needs of me and my family. But I had come too far and needed to finish the course.

I was placed on 9 weeks of 12.5 (full-time) night shifts on a busy obstetric-led Labour ward. I was not able to pump milk due to the workload (we were lucky to get a 30 minute break in a 12.5 hour shift) and I wasn't offered the opportunity or asked if I needed time to pump. I was not allowed to request day shifts. Sadly, and reluctantly, I ended up supplementing with formula while I was working - as pumping after night shifts, while trying to maintain breastfeeding and fit in some sleep during the day was impossible. My need to feed/pump was not even discussed when I returned - by either university or clinical practice areas. ***I was devastated that I was giving advice to women about feeding and pumping yet I wasn't supported to do the same and wasn't even asked****. My boobs would be engorged and painful by the end of each shift, and would leak heavily with each birth and every time a neonate cried."*

"As a qualified midwife I mostly worked in community but also worked for a short period of time in intrapartum areas.

In intrapartum areas, it was the norm to only have an unpaid 30 minute break in a 12.5 hour shift - despite only being paid for 11.5 hours. The rest of our unpaid 60 minute break was handover time - in theory our 'break' was us leaving half an hour early at the end of the shift. In reality we rarely left half hour early, so the ***midwives are owed hours and hours of these unpaid half hours that have not been taken as breaks.*** *It was 'normal' to not get a break until 4-5pm when on a long day shift.*

In one low risk intrapartum area it was not unusual to have 3 midwives covering 7 birth rooms with no 'co-ordinator' or admin support outside of the rooms. It was difficult to get a break as you were looking after 2 women. We tried to ensure that each midwife had women in different stages of Labour/birth/postnatal states but sometimes that wasn't possible."

"Today I finished a shift at a large hospital. We were massively understaffed. Only 7 [midwives] +2 [support workers] on delivery suite for a day shift. The night shift was down to 14 midwives (across delivery suite, antenatal, maternity assessment centre and postnatal).

This week ***I've hugged a neonatal nurse coming off her shift and sobbing in the stair well as she 'can't keep on doing this'. I've witnessed a very lovely colleague sobbing on the postnatal ward as for the umpteenth time in the last few months the ward has been understaffed and absolutely full.*** *I witnessed a partner being vile to her about how slow we were to discharge his wife and ask to speak to the coordinator to complain about her. I saw that same midwife break down in front of the HoM who was doing a walk around, sobbing that she can't keep on going like this. The HoM's advice? "Maybe we should use community midwives and our MVP to get the word out how busy we are, to set expectations with women and* *families that discharges take time". What I took from that comment was, "let's use our staff to set the expectation that we have hardly any staff on this ward so nobody gets miffed that they have nobody to look after them".*

I've spoken to another wonderful colleague telling me that her team of 7 experienced midwives in community will soon be 2 as 5 are leaving in the next few weeks. They will be replaced by x2 NQMs who will also be working on delivery suite. Let that sink in, x2 fresh midwives will be filling in for 5 very experienced midwives whilst also trying to consolidate their learning on delivery suite.

***The whole system is on its knees. Women, babies, families and midwives are suffering. It's NOT good enough!** I can't imagine urology and oncology having to deal with this. But then, birthing people and midwives are conditioned and will accept suboptimal staffing and care. We have the maternity system that reflects our society as it is now. It needs to change!"*

*"I have worked for the NHS for 43 years firstly as a nurse and as a midwife for the last 30. I retired and returned as a B6 having been B7 for many years in many areas including setting up and running a birth unit. I have never known midwifery to be in such a state. Every shift I work is short staffed. Trying to support students is a challenge as what they see is a system that is failing. Management (having been there) I appreciate have a tough time too but from the shop floor it appears that all they are interested in is meeting targets and ticking boxes. One unit manager would not allow the B7 to close the unit when it was clearly unsafe (she did escalate and was supported by the hospital duty manager). Some managers do not appreciate the complexity or acuity of the workload and pile more and more on you within each shift, meaning that you are spread so thinly. I am a very positive and upbeat person and try to keep that spirit at work for my colleagues but most importantly for the women but **it breaks my heart to see my colleagues in tears and being reprimanded for failing to undertake CQC tasks like daily checking when we can barely cover the workload."***

"I have been a community midwife for the past 14 years at the same Trust that I trained in (and had my own babies at).

There are currently huge concerns by all clinical staff over the safety of care for all women and their babies and the impact of the current situation on staff well-being.

The introduction of the continuity of Carer (CoC) model alongside a large increase in birth rates since Covid-19 at our Trust is having a huge detrimental impact on the quality and safety of care provided for women and their babies (the complete opposite of the predicted and promised improved outcomes of CoC) and the physical and mental well-being of midwifery staff. The unit has been left so short of staff (e.g. today, 1 midwife, who is also the coordinator, to cover the Labour ward which usually runs on 7 midwives and also Coordinate the whole unit) and midwives being asked to attend higher risk homebirths alone, as a result of staff being taken to make up the teams and used in escalation. This then means that the unit is in escalation almost every single shift. To cover the 'missing' midwives, staff who have worked all day are then called in to also work all night meaning most midwives are working 20+ hours a day on a regular basis."

"When I qualified, I began working at a large trust. From the beginning there was absolutely no guidance. ***We were given zero support, the bare minimum of training which was mostly vague box ticking, and were expected to learn on the job with no supernumerary time. For my first 7 months as a midwife on the AN/PN ward I felt completely unsafe.*** *Just left to get on with it. There was never any chance of rotation - once you'd worked in that ward you never went back, so it was mainly NQMs, and to management we were just bodies on the shop floor.*

I'm a resilient person (though I hate that phrase and what it insinuates), but every shift was filled with dread and anxiety. I kept thinking surely it will get better, I'll feel more prepared, more confident. Somehow, I will learn to take only a few minutes for each task. The constant pressure was hideous. 10 women and 10 babies - 12. 5 hours - that's 37 minutes to give each individual everything they need during your shift. These are mostly high-risk patients. It's unfathomable.

I got used to checklists, defensive documentation and taking 1 solitary minute in the cupboard to cry because that's all I could spare. I felt awfully selfish taking 5 minutes for a break during a shift because I was keeping women waiting for the already late medication round. I prioritised tasks based on what was most likely to cause harm, because at least when you hand over you can tell them that nobody died. Women were brought up fresh from an ELCS (elective caesarean section) without even a verbal handover. There was no such thing as breastfeeding support. I'd walk out of a bay after finally completing the nonsensically long discharge process, the woman beside herself with fury at being kept waiting, and within 2 minutes there was somebody new in the bed. It was impossible to do a discharge quickly as every 2 minutes the buzzer would go, and there was nobody else to answer it. Your 10 women and 10 babies are yours. The 2 support workers aren't free. ***Their lives are in your hands and whatever happens is on you. The guilt walking out feeling you had let everyone down was unbelievable."***

"I'm retired now, but I'm still extremely interested in the profession that I worked in all my career. I thought that since you're talking about a horrific series of events that were a little while ago, I'd just add that a few years ago, an old colleague of mine had a very similar experience. She actually wrote on the patient's notes/ partogram that she was 'exercising her accountability' and was too tired to continue any longer, and that as a professional she had to put the woman first. The coordinator was simply furious, but because she'd written in the notes, including the reason behind her comments... i.e. the long day she'd already worked, called in on the way home etc with no food etc, also including the fact that it was by then 01:00hrs ... the coordinators hands were tied. She was invited into the HoM's office several days later but there was nothing she could say either. This was a very quiet, timid midwife who just had had enough.... felt unsafe etc. etc. all the things we all knew and had felt at one time or another. It was never mentioned again and ironically, they never tried it again with her either.

One of the Trust solicitors at a study day I attended not long after said they could never defend defensive practice successfully, but they could defend the truth... or something similar..... I'm sure you will understand what he meant.

What's sad is that this was a few years ago ..., and apparently, it's still happening.... too much."

***"4 years qualified and have considered leaving the profession now more than ever.** Sometimes I feel like the joy is gone for me. I'm sick of feeling like I can't provide the care I want to provide (and the care that the people in my care deserve). I'm so tired of feeling like just another number in the conveyor belt that has become maternity services in the UK. Nothing feels woman centred anymore, it just feels like we're playing a numbers game. I have good days and bad days, but the only thing keeping me here is knowing I'm a bloody good midwife...but it's eventually going to come at a cost to my own mental/physical health. I have a great team leader and colleagues, but I feel like we're all just working in a system that's working directly against us. **It's sad, but 4 years in (and at the grand old age of 26) I shouldn't be dreaming about retirement**...the anti-social hours, poor pay and ever-increasing workload is making me consider a career move...but I'm holding out, hoping it gets better before it gets worse."*

"The accounts of community midwives being overworked are very familiar, frequently expected to work all day then be at a home birth all night. Being escalated into the unit without any thought of how this impacts the midwives or the families they care for. Hospital midwives would not be allowed to work for so long as it would be considered unsafe, so why is it ok for CMWs? I once worked a day

of postnatal visits, then straight to a home birth, then there was nobody to relieve me to do all the immediate postnatal work, ***so I worked 27 hrs straight. How I didn't crash my car driving home I'll never know."***

"Nobody ever helps community out as it's considered non-urgent. All the time the to-do list is getting longer, and it is women and families (including the midwives) that suffer. Birthrate+ says we are appropriately staffed so our HoM isn't recruiting. We are absolutely not safely staffed. The amount we are expected to do in an antenatal check is growing all the time. I have handed my notice in because I can't tolerate these working conditions or the thought that I can't provide safe care."

"The management have been told time and time again about the concerns from multiple staff members, including the band 7 shift leads who raised concerns as a group to the Trust Board. Maternity management and the LMNS are so focused on having the best statistics for CoC that they are ignoring the warning signs and pushing through another 2 teams no matter what the consequences are. It has been escalated to the Trust board and CEO but still it continues as I don't believe they have a true vision of what is happening on a day-to-day basis. We have a matron and a HOM who could 'sell sand to the Sahara' so always seem to be able to manage to convince the board that everything is fine.

The homebirth team which has been running successfully for many years is now being disbanded and divided amongst the teams. This is not only devastating for them and the service users but extremely unsafe. This week alone, a traditional community midwife who has not been the lead in delivery for several years, was sent to a homebirth for a high-risk woman with a CoC midwife who had never done a homebirth since being a student. She had no confidence and was petrified. The other midwife felt extremely uneasy with the situation. We are being constantly put into situations which make us feel out of our depth and it's so dangerous.

The theory is that the CoC midwives will also be doing their own homebirths on top of covering shifts in the unit.

Don't get me wrong, CoC in theory is lovely of course, but in reality, there are just not enough staff for it to run safely and effectively.

The evidence for the CoC model shows that there are better outcomes for women and babies...this is absolutely not the case as it stands. In fact, it is a disaster waiting to happen.

In addition, the Women are also not actually receiving 'continuity'. The way the teams work, a woman may actually see several midwives throughout her pregnancy and be delivered by another who she may have never met, but because it's 'one of the team' it counts as continuity! That completely contradicts the whole ethos behind continuity of Carer. The concerns regarding the sustainability and efficacy of CoC as well as the well-being of staff are echoed in the written evidence from the maternity review panel/Donna Ockenden which seems to have gone completely ignored.

I truly fear that it will take the death of a woman, a midwife or both to get management's heads out of the sand and stop this utter destruction of our maternity services. *I'm desperate for the CQC or other outside agencies to get involved and stop this before yet again we are 'learning from our mistakes."*

"Institutional toxicity is going to be so hard to change."

"I love my core labour ward role and I love having and teaching students. *I help out at uni skills sessions and interviews. Because I love teaching and moulding our new cohorts of future colleagues I do so from a place of positive nurturing and encouragement within the professional guidance of our Code. However, recently, like many others,* ***I find myself tired stressed and burnt out.*** *Struggling to give the best care to patients. I often feel I've not done enough to the standard I expect from myself. Add to this the constant evaluation, assessment, teaching and mentoring of students, it's just too much. Now, if I feel I don't have the capacity to teach students as they deserve and just scrape the bare minimum, we will be churning out 'only just passed' NQM who will struggle. This lets them down and our profession but most importantly our service users. Under par NQM is hard to recover from, we will be forever struggling and will see more poor service user experience. For those who dislike teaching and only do the bare minimum to pass on to the next mentor to deal with, add into those the exhaustion, students really have no hope. I can already see toxic attitudes in 2nd & 3rd year students being displayed as that is the environment, they are learning in. They think this is normal. And it's wrong and toxic and needs to change from the ground up. I also feel the standards set for training are inadequate. Currently they have to either pass or fail a semester. I have two students at the moment. Both passed their first year, but one is far more suited to the role and beyond her knowledge for a new 2nd year than the other student who only just scraped a pass, and can barely grasp the job! yet on paper, it appears they are the same level, which they absolutely are not! Everyone is being let down, Staff, students and this impacts service users. We have to stop breeding toxicity into the students as they will teach that to newer students and in their own* *teaching when qualified, delivering substandard care because they 'passed' but only by the skin of their teeth, rather than a well-deserved and well-earned flying colours pass!"*

"Being pulled from my contracted area of work and having my job role as a low risk, core, birth centre midwife changed almost every shift and moved to work in high-risk areas of midwifery that I hadn't worked in for 6 years, with no support and just expected to 'slot in' get on with it and be expected to know the guidelines, and the way the ward runs and be competent, confident and provide safe care. Being pulled to be a NIPE (Newborn and Infant Physical Examination) midwife almost every shift. ***Turning up to work not knowing where I was going to be working****. Feeling like I was becoming de-skilled as a low-risk woman centred midwife as I never stayed in the area that provided low risk care. No sense of 'team' or 'belonging' as other midwives never took the time to get to know me as there was a big 'them and us' culture between low-risk birth centre and the high-risk area, and midwives were in some areas very busy and had no time for a break let alone getting to know each other. Working regularly without a break, or quickly eating between auscultations, with no proper rest.* ***The expectation that I can work 12.5 hours on just 30 mins break (if I was lucky) when I was entitled to 1 hour's unpaid break.*** *Escalated concerns about not feeling competent on other wards, and lack of support falling on deaf ears. Having to cut corners and provide care which did not marry with my morals, or beliefs and which I believed was substandard due to staff shortages and ratio of work to midwives. Poor management support and lack of professionalism from managers. Window of normality for women getting smaller and smaller, more women being induced, more risk factors introduced increasing fear in women and the recommendation to birth on obstetric led. Bullying from some doctors and band 7 managers in high-risk areas when decisions questioned. Lack of autonomy. Huge blame culture in the trust. Inability to engage with and listen to staff."*

"I have just left my job as Continuity of Carer Midwife as even working 70 hours a week wasn't enough! *My boss was a yes person (to management…which makes sense why someone with no experience was promoted into the role).* ***I would tell her that I was working to breaking point and she would just say we work to get the job done, not the number of hours!*** *I never got paid a penny of overtime, I was told to join the bank…but I have no capacity to do extra hours.* ***I asked for my time back in lieu and never got a response. That's why I have left.*** *I am taking time out then will return.* ***As for bullying, it is awful! It does vary from trust to trust, but it's a pandemic all of its own!*** *For a profession that is focused on supporting women, some midwives are unable to see that we should be supporting each other too!"*

Burnout/Exhaustion

These accounts clearly illustrate the outcomes of a midwifery system that does not value and is not listening to midwives. There are clear examples of bullying by colleagues and an expectation that the work gets done with little or no compassion for colleagues who have worked all day and are expected to work additional hours to cover other service areas, leading to exhaustion and burnout and considering leaving or having left the profession they love.

"I've been a midwife for only 6 years which I feel is still relatively new. ***I had a breakdown with absolute exhaustion and burnout.*** *I'm a community midwife and we regularly are called to labour ward for cover of staff shortages after a full day at work.* ***My colleagues and I will only be home an hour to be told to be there at the start of the night shift.*** *And then when we ask to leave (because we feel unsafe to practice) we are scoffed at and told "well don't you think I am tired too?!" Or* ***we are excluded from the "staff pizza" order and whilst they're all sitting there living their best lives,*** *we are working our backsides off looking after labourer after labourer, like we are being penalised for being a community midwife. It's frankly abuse.*

I don't sleep properly at night knowing that one of our team will have been called out all night. And knowing the impact it'll have on the following day covering their work as well as clinics and the extra visits and then it continues the next night and the night after that.

I don't want to be a midwife right now. I was getting to the point of just ticking boxes and doing the bare essentials to get through each day. I've been signed off work. I'm not sure how much time I'll need because something desperately needs to change as I'll go back to the same rubbish and will burn out again. I know a couple of my colleagues are at breaking point and admire those that are so resilient. But I also know if this systematic abuse of community midwives continues there will be walk outs and it'll take one fatal mistake for one of us to be hauled over the coals and be blamed and penalised. ***We are tired."***

"I am a continuity of care midwife, have been qualified for four years now as feel confident both in and out of the unit. I don't ever mind helping labour ward and always feel supported when I'm called in. However, ***I recently have had to take two weeks off due to work place stress and exhaustion. I was regularly working 50-60 hours on call a month on top of my usual full-time hours.*** *We work 8-4 and then on call from 8:30-8am overnight. Supposed to be only called to care for our caseload, but usually it's for escalation. Every night on call is essentially a night shift. You wouldn't be able to book an early shift and a night on the same day, but it's acceptable for CofC? I regularly work 20 hours, with no break. Labour ward often only has 2/3 core midwives per shift, including the "supernumerary" midwife in charge.* ***Our CofC teams, pretty much staff the labour ward to make us up to full numbers. Often, we are given 13 hour shifts straight after on calls. So, you go home at 8am and you're back the same morning for a long day.***

I love continuity of care, and in an ideal world, where staffing is adequate, it works really well for me and is the model I'd like to work in. But the constant working for escalation is demoralising.

It affects our caseload care because it means we are often short due to our midwives being out overnight. We have to give visits to other teams and traditional model as we can't manage it ourselves. This defeats the point of continuity.

Luckily, I've realised management at my workplace are supportive of us. The band 7s on labour ward always apologise for calling us in, what else can they do? The answer is "we are getting new preceptors etc" but how long until they are broken too?

I have made serious errors at work due to tiredness. We always escalate when we feel unsafe, however if there is no one to physically relieve you, everyone is already in the unit that they can call, how can you just go home?

I really do hope this issue is resolved because I love midwifery and can't imagine working anywhere else but am considering leaving every day."

"One of the most significant times of a woman's life is entrusted to us, and we are expected to treat people as though they are on a conveyor belt - numbers, bodies, problems to be solved and removed as fast as possible. I couldn't in good conscience keep going, ***and when I talked to a colleague about how I was feeling, I was told to 'lower my expectations'****. One day a manager did ask how I was - I*

told her I was finding it really difficult and not coping. She just smile
walked away."

"We have so many midwives off with work related stress due to burn out (for example, 3 of the CoC teams of 8 has only 2 working members as the other 6 are off with stress) this obviously has an impact on the remaining staff and ultimately the quality of care provided. The community staff who are left to cover the traditional model of care is now so depleted that there is frequently only one midwife (sometimes none with multiple clinics uncovered) available to provide postnatal home visits for the whole of the local area and surrounding villages (around 60 mile Radius). We have 8 midwives to provide AN/PN care and homebirth on calls for the remaining 60% of the birthing population (approximately 4000 births). There's a constant 'begging' for staff to do extra shifts on their days off to cover clinics and postnatal visits. CoC midwives are having to do bank hours on top of their full-time hours to facilitate their antenatal care for their women."

"I volunteered to join a new CoC team and was eager for it to work as I was a firm believer in the concept. *However, I lasted less than 6 months before begging to come back and work in the core. It was this or leave the profession completely.*

Despite working part time, my caseload was twice the number it should have been. *Each week I was asked to do another task/offer support/be available for other teams: eventually leaving less time for my caseload.*

The flexibility I was promised in CoC did not exist, only 1 member of the team is left working in this model everyone else has left. I was working several days a week alongside a day and night on call each week. Due to staffing shortages, I was called at least once a week to work for escalation. It didn't matter if I had already worked my contracted hours.

I loved the relationships with my caseload and for those with vulnerabilities really saw the benefit of my care. However, I only ever cared for 1 woman on my caseload in labour; of the others I cared for under my team I had only met 2 prior to labour.

Working in this way broke me, I struggled to cope with the constant switch from nights to days. *The anxiety of waiting to be called in and inability to plan or do things with my life stopped me from seeing my family. I felt like I failed at midwifery asking to come back to the core however I had to priorities my own health and well-being."*

"I feel like I have survivor's guilt. Our 2 continuity teams have barely any midwives doing on calls (so how is it continuity) because they were abused so much to cover gaps in the unit. I am concerned about the push for continuity by March 2023. Where will these midwives come from? Regularly as bleep holder I was faced with 50% staffing. I was tired of being shouted at by staff because they had been pushed to the edge. ***I left in September and cannot believe the difference now in education. I hadn't realised how burnt out I was.*** *I am so sad for midwifery."*

Resilience

These accounts highlight the resentment felt by midwives when the solution presented for all problems is to be more resilient and to have better workload management skills.

"I detest the word resilience. It has become short hand for suck it up and continue to be disrespected."

"The current state of maternity services is shocking. No wonder you are broken. The severe shortage of staff impacts on everyone, & of course the care we can give. Not helped by unsympathetic/lack of support from management. I feel things have been heading this way for several years. I retired, after over 40 years given to the NHS in 2018 so missed out on the added stress of working during the Covid pandemic. ***I despise that word "resilient", so frequently used when staff are struggling to cope with an impossible workload. I remember being told to "man up" when asking for more staff."***

"This is so depressing in some ways but also illuminating knowing none of us are the only one. I didn't realize how widespread these experiences are ***and the feeling of shame we all carry for lack of that nebulous "resilience"****. Everyone has a breaking point and years ago we were there, now it feels like we're all broken but terrified of quitting because what would happen to the clients without even the broken staff?"*

"It feels like a domestic abuse relationship being a midwife at the moment."

On Call

While historically it is recognised that on-call rotas are necessary to provide some maternity care services in the community, for example, planned home births, the purpose of the on-call has changed over the years and is often used to prop up an obstetric unit with little or no thought of the impact on the community services or care providers. Frequently the on-call is covered by community midwives who may be less experienced and familiar with acute intrapartum care. On-calls have increasingly impacted on their community workload, including working additional excessive hours leading to concerns about safe care and the well-being of the midwife.

"Having experience the issues of working all day driving over 50 miles on visits and clinics then getting home at 6pm, out at 7pm homebirth which was a 75 mile round trip on country lanes all night having to return home, being made to feel guilty for refusing to run my antenatal clinic my argument saying I wasn't safe and having to drive another 20 miles home, who would be responsible if I crashed? ***I cried all the way home. Again, working a 12 hour shift being begged to either go on a 5 to 6 hour transfer or stay on the unit till the transfer got back.*** *When you are running on 5's what can you do?"*

"In our trust the Community Midwives have a split on call rota, before Midnight and from Midnight. Both are awful. If you are before Midnight, you can start work at 8 and be called into the Unit, (or a home birth) work all night until the midnight arrives (they have travel time to get to you so may be 1230/0100 plus hand over time. If they are sent to relieve you, you can go home.

You have then have a small window of sleep until you have to get up and work your normal working day. For the second on call, you have got home after usually a 10 hour day with no break and little to drink and tried to go to bed early as you know you need some sleep, in case you are called out.

You lie there willing sleep. Russian roulette!

Will I be called out? Maybe get an hour or two if you are lucky or wake frequently in the night waiting for a call. If called for unit you may work all night with no break and then either carry on and cover your clinic and visits or go home for a few hours' sleep as it is expected for you to work sometime that day. For home births we are first on call for our area and second Midwife for another area which can involve travelling 45 minutes to 90 minutes to get there.

It's not just the working that is unsafe but the travelling.

It's terrifying. *Worse in the winter as these are sometimes ungritted country roads.*

The Trust get out clause now is that it is our responsibility to say no but the bullying and repercussions for saying no is immense."

"I have been a midwife for 9 years. 7.5 years in community. Which is the only reason I'm still a midwife. Community is real midwifery. Homebirth, antenatal care, decent post-natal care. Making a huge difference to the women in your care. Until we merged.... ***Now we were managed by a ruthless management team. Saving money, saving hours. At our expense.*** *Midwives started leaving. On calls for CMW now expanding across our old borders. Travelling up to 1.5 hrs at the max to get to a HB. We used to have compensatory rest. Out for 6 hrs, get 6 hrs in bed etc. Now....oh no! Now we owe any hours we sleep the next day. So, if you're full time you are expected to use your time owing. What time owing? All those missed lunches and getting off late now has to be recorded. If we don't have any time owing then we have to work an extra shift to pay back the hours.*

No one cares if you have an awful off duty. One full time week includes a weekend and so then rolls into the following week. Possibly 9 days straight with 2 on calls. Being called out twice, not just HB but to support the unit. In fact, now it's more often to support the unit. HB service was cancelled through August and September and we were consistently called in overnight. One midwife had 4 on calls in 9 days and when she said she couldn't do that, she was dismissed and told it's on her off duty and that's that. ***She pleaded saying she couldn't cope with that. They just dismissed her pleas.***

Another staff member has had one set day off for the last 2 years. But because no flexible working was in place, they changed her off duty. ***Told her to submit a flexible working request which she did and they denied it! She is now considering leaving due to childcare issues."***

"Midwives work bank on their AL to cover their clinics. Because there is no staff to do it. *Request to reduce hours is denied. Because it cannot work in the current service. Midwives do not want to come out to community because they see what is being done to us. We have not started CoC yet due to our appalling staffing levels. If we do, when we do....I fear for those midwives left. We mostly run a community service on part time midwives now. COC can't work with that off duty and no staff. I don't know where we go from here. But will continually strive for change...for the better."*

"Midwives in tears feeling they're pretty much guaranteed to be called in overnight but they're supposed to be on a back-to-back clinic the following day *and there's no one to cover it meaning they'll end up trying to squash them in another day when they were going to do bookings/ chase bloods. They then end up chasing bloods and responding to emails whilst half asleep or in the evenings as 'when else can they do it'. When they're called in and don't work the following* *day, they still owe those hours. If you're full time that basically means the more, you're called in the less days off you have. Midwives opting to work bank during their annual leave because there's no one to cover their clinics and the women still need seeing. Midwives not opting to work bank during annual leave but subsequently dreading the time off and feeling anxious the whole time off about the work that's backing up while they're off or equally exhausted because they've had to work extra to 'clear the decks' prior to annual leave. Last weekend there was 1 community midwife on for the whole of the city each day as the other one (only 2 rostered in the first place) was called into the unit overnight having worked all day plus overtime to get visits seen. The overtime doesn't count towards the on call so they can still be brought in for their full allowance. Sunday the Manager on call then gave permission for that 1 midwife to go out to a homebirth as, in her own words' she didn't really understand how community works and didn't realise it would be an issue'. 1 midwife already seeing women in clinic plus has visits to do and also no 2nd on call as back up. They're also having to run new patient clinics in order to see more women than visits would allow meaning we're dragging back in poor women who maybe were only discharged the evening before. They are then the ones having to apologise to these exhausted and in pain women who go onto social media to berate their community midwives when the reason there isn't someone to see them at home is that they were working overnight in the unit."*

"In community, the on-call policy was to have two midwives on call for homebirths and to potentially come into the unit in escalation. There was also a 'reserve' in case of sickness. On a number of occasions, I was the reserve (made up to on call) or designated on call alone. I was advised there were no other community midwives to be on call with me so rather than cancelling the on-call service that night - I was told to ask if one of the unit night shift midwives could come with me if called out. With no guarantee that they would/could or who it would even be, expression of concern was not met positively and dismissed.

When called in to cover the unit we would be told to go home and sleep and come in at 10pm or midnight and work through until 8am, having already worked a full 8am-6pm day in community. *It was expected that we would staff a busy ward (20+ beds) or be an extra body on the high-risk labour ward. Again, regardless of skills/confidence/experience in those areas.* ***If concern was raised it was dismissed and would be negatively viewed as the midwife being obstructive and putting women at risk by not turning up.*** *This was to avoid closing beds and diverting women to other units. Calling one or two community midwives into the unit or out on homebirths had a significant impact on the next day's community workload as rather than being paid for the time called out, the time was taken back* *the next working day. This was good as you could sleep, but meant clinics/visits either needed covering by the remaining community midwives or were cancelled and rearranged.*

The suggestion was made that unit staff should have an on-call system in place to cover in hospital areas - that was dismissed as unit staff 'don't do on-calls'. ***This made community staff feel less valued as our health/time/sleep/day to day workload was less important."***

"The longest shift I ever did was 26 hours. I worked 8am-6pm in community (clinics and visits), then as I pulled into my driveway at home at 7pm I was called to a homebirth, we went to the unit following the homebirth at 6am to submit documentation and return equipment/clinical waste and were immediately called to a BBA. We then didn't leave after going back out to deal with this until 10:30am the next day. I managed to reverse into a bollard leaving the car park and felt drunk driving home - I still have no idea of the actual route I drove. I must've driven on autopilot.

Another time I had been awake most of the night before a shift with sick children. I called in on the morning of my shift/on call to say I needed to take parental leave as my kids were really poorly with high temps and I hadn't had any sleep. I was told I could take the day but I still needed to cover the on call. I explained again I'd had no sleep for over 24 hours and couldn't do it, could the reserve cover? Nope - the reserve had no childcare. I said I didn't feel safe to cover the on call especially if I was called in to cover the unit. ***I tried to escalate and went to a union rep. Unfortunately, I was told I had to do it, the unsaid implication being it would be a disciplinary matter if I didn't.*** *I cried and cried so much that day, because my kids were sick, I was exhausted, I didn't feel safe or cared for or supported. I had no one to turn to.*

Luckily my kind colleague consoled exhausted me, crying me on the phone, and collected me from home in her car when we were called out to a homebirth - she was concerned I wasn't safe to drive. She was disgusted I had been made to cover it and told me she would take the lead. We were out all night; ***I had not slept already for 30 hours at the time we were called out and I was absolutely exhausted.*** *Luckily the homebirth was a straight forward one and my colleague took the lead, I was running on caffeine and sugar. I finally got home to sleep after being awake for pretty much three days - (e.g. I slept Mon night, worked Tues, didn't sleep because poorly kids Tues night, called in Weds morning and facilitated the homebirth Weds night. I finally slept during the day after getting home on the Thursday morning!).* ***This event pretty much cemented my desire to leave clinical midwifery. I knew at that point I was just a body and not cared for, and easily replaced."***

"I work 9-5, have a filled day but frequently expected to rearrange my work to work in the unit - then get complaints that my work isn't done! On calls we are called into the unit for 4 hours - the policy - but ends up more. ***Bully culture is "you'll do as you're told". After 30 years as a midwife, I'm ready to leave.*** *I'm petrified I'll make a mistake or crash driving. It leaves community constantly short. There is the assumption that we sit drinking tea all day. We were the last to be considered during covid despite going into homes where numbers weren't controlled despite no visiting in hospital. I feel so let down."*

"I'm a traditional community midwife and qualified 4 years ago. We currently do on calls for homebirth and often get called into the unit as well. We work 10 hour shifts (8-6pm) and then the on call is from 6pm -8am, we don't get to go home early or rest before our on-call starts and more often than not we are still out on visits or in the office doing admin when it starts. Many of us live a good hour away as well. If we get called out, we are still expected to work the next day and if we don't, we are told we owe a shift. ***We were told by HR that we needed to be more "resilient" when we raised the concerns of basically working 34 hours straight!!*** *Our community teams are so short staffed we are running on 4 midwives instead of 7/8 with no help from the hospital. If a member of our team calls in sick it's left to us to cover the on-call despite having done our own (sometimes 2 a week) and having child care to arrange etc. Staff that have temporary health issues and can't do on calls are threatened to move back into the hospital, one staff member was even told not to take her medication once a week so that she could be on call.* ***We get Zero help or support from management. It's honestly so bad at the moment, everyone is leaving or going sick and the morale is just so low. I've seen strong midwives basically beaten into submission where they now just accept whatever is thrown at them for fear of being bullied!*** *It's horrendous! Let's hope we can change things; we are losing good midwives at an alarming rate."*

"This was about 6/7 years ago when I was working in community and my first day back after AL, I had my AN clinic and was night on call. Before my leave I'd blocked out appointments from 3pm with a note to say I was on call for whomever was covering the clinic. When I returned, I was gobsmacked that appointments had been scheduled up until 5:30pm - later than a normal clinic day - and squeezed into my lunch break! I'd spoken to my team leader to see if anyone could cover the later appointments, nope. I tried to get hold of women to reschedule to later in the week, didn't manage many calls due to the clinic being busy. I didn't get home until 7:20pm and was on call from 8pm. Shortly after 8 I was called into labour ward. I'd literally just inhaled "lunch" before setting off.

I was looking after a woman having augmentation, happy coincidence, it was someone from my clinic so familiar with her, her partner and her history.

It got to 11pm and I went to ask for a break, coordinator told me there wasn't anyone to relieve me and as the woman was on Syntocinon needed continuous 1:1 care.

Shortly after 1am I felt like I was about to collapse, when I went out the Manager on call (who also happened to be the Head of Midwifery) was coordinating.

I asked for break relief. 'No.'

I said I require a break as I am the CMW who got called in. 'No - no one has had a break.'

I said unlike everyone else on shift, I NEED a break because I have worked all day before coming in. "So have I".

"With all due respect HoM, I have worked clinically 9-6, not at a desk, without a lunch break and was at home less than an hour before coming in to provide 1:1 care. I am unsafe and I am telling you I am going for a break or I'm leaving."

The HoM then agreed I could have 20 minutes and she would pop in to check on my woman!

I cried for that time.

The shift continued and at 5am I was told I'd shortly be relieved to go home. I was relieved but then was told I needed to attend a homebirth as a second midwife to a "difficult woman" and was also told I have a duty to support any birthing woman as well as my colleague. At that point I'd lost all fight and I got a taxi to the homebirth and cried the entire journey.

I'd never met the first midwife before, but as soon as I arrived, she informed me that the woman is "non-compliant" with an "obstructive doula" and I need to take over. I calmly informed her I've been on LW all night and was there to support her not take over.

Anyway, I tiptoed into the birthing room with my finger over my lips to indicate I wasn't going to disturb anyone. The woman, her partner and doula were lovely, just wanted their plans and environment respected. We chatted about monitoring, surges, plans, she requested a VE...no obstruction whatsoever. I was gobsmacked when it hit 8am and the first midwife was at the door with her coat on saying her shift had ended and as this wasn't her area she was leaving. Yes, I reported this but don't believe there were any consequences. I was relieved at 8:50am. Had an hour long journey home and was asleep within minutes of getting home.

I woke up in the evening with severe abdominal and back pain. It was then I realised that I'd not had a drink in over 24hours and hadn't passed urine since the previous morning! This physical impact on my body really shook me.

I escalated all my concerns and was thanked for my resilience. I detest that word.

Insult to injury, apparently e-roster couldn't be overridden to state I'd effectively worked 08:30-08:30 with an hour at home. So, my team leader said I had to make do with what was rota-ed and I should've left earlier because I had a clinic the following day.

I've never had a shift like it since, but sadly I hear and read similar accounts more frequently now."

"There is little understanding from the Unit that you have worked all day and have had little or no sleep. ***Community is seen as a soft option by some Unit Midwives and a place where we don't really 'work'.*** *There is no acknowledgement that we have already been working all day. When one of us has a serious car accident or makes a serious mistake, who will be to blame? Yes, us not the trust. This is not new and there is no one to help protect us. We love working with the women and families but we are becoming more and more broken and leaving. The circle continues, less staff more pressure."*

"This seems to be the sad reality of community based midwifery, ***we are just seen as a source of cannon fodder for inpatient services.*** *This will only stop when we reclaim community from 'integrated teams' and ensure that all areas are properly staffed and we are given the respect that we deserve."*

"I've left 3 times, each time returning thinking it may have changed. But no.

I felt that midwives were no longer treated as autonomous practitioners, but harbingers of policies and protocols set up to protect the authorities.

Unrealistic expectations were heaped on midwives. *Trying to care for too many mums at once whilst facilitating a learning environment for others. Covering for staff shortages, extended shifts, no breaks, little support.*

Days off became recovery time, wondering what would happen next, if there were any repercussions from the last shift, if you could have done better. From wanting ideal outcomes for others, you suddenly realise it's unachievable given the situations we are in, and you need to look after yourself.

Bullying was also a factor in my first break from midwifery, stemming from non-work-related issues. I felt it was unprofessional to allow outside factors to influence your work practices to the point where you set others up to fail, yet no one cared.

In the end, after much soul searching, I realised my learning and expertise belonged to me! I could do what I wanted with it and use it where it was appreciated! Which I did, was like a breath of fresh air! My experience has not left me unscathed, but it will not prevent me from supporting women and families in an area I'm passionate about."

"Eventually the stress, overwhelm and relentlessness was too much. I had a breakdown and got sent home. Panic attacks, vertigo and insomnia were my way of life and looking back I'm so sad I kept going that long (for £12/hr, no less). *I moved to a small unit where I'm much happier. Things aren't perfect, but the difference is marked. I have palpitations whenever I talk about my first job and I genuinely can't believe midwives continue working that way. My colleagues at that first trust kept me going and were truly incredible people, my heart aches for them. Lots have left but so many keep on grafting.*

Continuity of carer is being painted as the enemy at the moment, but for me, without this way of working I don't think I could be a midwife any longer. To do things properly you need time. A smaller caseload. Flexibility. More bloody staff. I want the women I care for to feel that they matter to me, they are not just a number. It's difficult, yes, and draining - mixed shifts and on calls aren't for everyone. But there has to be a better way than how things are currently. It's simply not good enough for women, babies, families, midwives, or anyone. I know I am idealistic, but I steadfastly refuse to 'lower my expectations' about the care that women deserve. I'm so glad we are finally hearing the true accounts of modern midwifery and desperately hope something can be done to save our profession."

The accounts within this section speak for themselves and need no further explanation. They are heart wrenchingly powerful and reflect the reality for some midwives and the effects on midwifery staff: - exhaustion, burnout and despair. Many midwives have now left the profession because of the way they have been treated when they report their workload as too difficult and unsafe. They have reported feeling bullied into accepting the situation and advised to increase their resilience, which is unhelpful, victim blaming and does not address the cause of their distress. Midwives need compassionate support when their expected workloads exceed their capacity and the maternity service needs to address the factors that cause this distress.

Becky Millar
Nurse, RN, Midwife, RM, BSc Nursing (Adult), BSc Midwifery, MSc Advanced Practice Student

References

Dharni, N. Essex, H. Bryant, A. Cronin de Chavez, K. Farrar, D. Bywater, T. Dickerson, J. (2021) The key components of a successful model of midwifery-led continuity of carer, without continuity at birth: findings from a qualitative implementation evaluation. BMC Pregnancy and Childbirth 21(1)

Kirkup, B. (2015) The Report of the Morecambe Bay Investigation. The Stationary Office. London

McInnes, R. Aitken-Arbuckle, A. Lake, S. Hollins Martin, C & Juliet MacArthur, J. (2020) Implementing continuity of midwife carer – just a friendly face? A realist evaluation. BMC Health Services Research. 20, (304)

NHS England (2016) National Maternity Review. Better Births. Improving outcomes of maternity services in England. A Five Year Forward View for Maternity Care. Downloaded from **www.england.nhs.uk/wp-content/uploads/2016/02/national-maternity-review-report.pdf**

NHS Resolution (2021) Maternity Incentive Scheme. Downloaded from **www.resolution.nhs.uk/services/claims-management/clinical-schemes/clinical-negligence-scheme-for-trusts/maternity-incentive-scheme**

NMC (2018) The Code. Professional standards of practice and behaviour for nurses, midwives and nursing associates. Nursing and Midwifery Council. London.

The Nursing and Midwifery Board of Ireland. (2022). Practice Standard for Midwives. 2nd ed. 18/20 Carysfort Avenue: Blackrock, Dublin: NMBI.pp. 11-13. Board of Scottish Government, (2017)

The best start: five-year plan for maternity and neonatal care. **www.gov.scot/publications/best-start-five-year-forward-plan-maternity-neonatal-care-scotland**

Stephenson, J. (2020) Heads of midwifery warn over staffing and recruitment problems. Nursing Times. **www.nursingtimes.net/news/workforce/heads-of-midwifery-warn-over-safe-staffing-and-recruitment-problems-03-03-2020**

Taylor B, Cross-Sudworth F, Goodwin L, Kenyon S, MacArthur C, (2019) Midwives perspectives of continuity based working in the UK: A cross-sectional survey. Midwifery. Vol 74 pp 127-137.

Walton, G. (2021) RCM warns of midwife exodus as maternity staffing crisis grows. **www.rcm.org.uk/media-releases/2021/september/rcm-warns-of-midwife-exodus-as-maternity-staffing-crisis-grows/**

Chapter 4:
Why Midwives Leave?

"Someone needs to stop people feeling like me and other midwives do, all we wanted was to go to work and do a good job"

Becoming a registered midwife is often a long-held dream and one that is achieved through hard work, resilience, a commitment, and passion to provide quality care for women and babies. It also comes at a cost; financially for the commissioning body/organisation or the individual if self-funding- often with many personal and family sacrifices on the way. There is increasing awareness that given the nature of maternity care services, a range of 'Human Factors' such as stress, fatigue, and pressure can contribute to errors that impact on the care provided to women (Royal College of Midwives, 2021). Reports in the media, the literature, and the accounts below, highlight that when subjected to bullying, being a student midwife or a midwife comes at a high cost, in terms of health and wellbeing, job loss, financial hardship, stress, self-harm and in some cases, suicide.

Bullying is a workplace phenomenon, with psychological and physical behaviours that can be likened to domestic abuse. The first description of the phenomenon is attributed to Heinemann (1972) and focused on bullying in schools. Adams (1992) was one of the first authors to write about bullying in the workplace with Scandinavian authors (Einarsen and Skogstad, 1996; Leyman, 1996; Vartia 1996; Niedl) 1996 reporting on the phenomenon in the mid 1990's. At the same time, in the UK, the Health Service Unions were among the first organisations to examine bullying in the workplace (Royal College of Midwives 1996, UNISON 1997, Royal College of Nurses (2002). Ball, Curtis and Kirkham (2002) identified that a large minority of respondents in their Why do Midwives Leave (WML) study had experienced bullying and or horizontal violence from their colleagues or managers, with little support forthcoming and often a sense that this behaviour was condoned.

Since those early days of research into workplace bullying, the body of literature on this workplace phenomenon continues to grow, both within and outside of the profession of midwifery. Consistently, the literature reports on the harm that is caused to individuals and organisations. While conflict in the workplace is normal and healthy, with constructive challenge and feedback important in an innovative and evolving work environment, workplace bullying is a complex phenomenon, with three attributes that help differentiate it from other poor working relationships. Bullying tends to be a repeated behaviour (one-off behaviours are not as impactful), difficult to defend against (usually due to a power differential) and has a negative impact on the target of bullying (Gillen et al., 2004, 2008). The intent of the bully is also an interesting element of the bullying phenomenon, with researchers' undecided about the intent of the bully and whether or not intent matters- it is the impact of the behaviour on the target that matters most.

To fully understand the concept of bullying, it is important also to consider the antecedents to bullying, as they are an event or condition that must occur, prior to bullying taking place and as such, it may be possible to alter these to reduce or minimise bullying (Walker and Avant, 2005; Gillen, 2008). Perception is important, as a target of bullying, the perception of a behaviour as bullying is key. Also, a lack of control is important. Midwives often work within a hierarchical environment with limited control and autonomy, leading to frustration, which may lead to bullying of those over whom they have some control e.g. student midwives or a less experienced/ newer member of staff. The third antecedent is power distance, which in essence is the use of interpersonal power or influence between individuals, with the person with the most power and control, using this power imbalance to bully the target. Lastly, the culture within which midwives work is a contributory factor to bullying in midwifery with the culture being viewed as permissive. Bullying behaviour is often ignored and therefore, a perception exists that it is allowed and even how one gets promoted. Where bullying is not tolerated, it is less like to happen. Leaders can make a huge difference by tackling bullying and not allowing it (Keller, Allie & Levine, 2019). Where bullying exists, understanding why is important and often particular to each workplace. Culture change and a commitment by organisations to undertake multidisciplinary resource-intensive interventions over a sustained period of time that optimise the working culture and minimise the potential for bullying are essential (Gillen et al., 2017; Nielsen & Einarsen, 2018).

Another aspect of bullying that is important to consider, is the role that witnesses or bystanders to the bullying behaviour, play. A witness observes or overhears someone being bullied with up to 83% witnessing bullying behaviour at some point (Chatziioannidis et al., 2017) An active bystander is someone who not only witnesses but takes steps to help the target or victim in some way. A typology of bystanders has been developed assigning labels and categorising the bystanders' actions or inactions as Destructive (unhelpful), Constructive (helpful) and Active or Passive (Paull, Omari and Standen, 2012) and range from those who support the bully to those who provide assistance, unwittingly or otherwise, to the target. Interestingly Mulder et al, (2017) report that most witnesses expect targets to confront the bully and whether or not they do this can be viewed positively or negatively by bystanders and may affect whether or not the bystander intervenes.

The Job Demand and Resource Model (Bakker & Denerouti, 2014) helps to further illuminate the role of the bystander as it explains how being bullied adds demand on the target and when failing to intervene, bystanders further add to that demand. When bystanders help the target, the bystander can serve as a resource for the target, reducing demand (Ng, Niven and Notelaers, 2022). The consequences of being subjected to bullying in midwifery are varied and impact at individual, professional and organisational level. Women are also affected as midwives who are bullies or are being bullied may not provide the high standard of compassionate care that women and babies deserve. Women also see and hear what is happening and this affects how safe and secure they feel. Maternity services and midwifery are chronically understaffed, and some would suggest that the stress of understaffing leads to further bullying, affecting recruitment and retention of staff. The recent Ockenden Report cites a culture of fear and bullying as a contributing factor to suboptimal care for women and babies (Ockenden, 2022).

This chapter includes accounts from midwives in the United Kingdom who have submitted a self-reported account of their bullying experience on the #saynotobullyinginmidwifery Facebook group. Some accounts and details (names/ places) have been removed where it was thought necessary, in order to protect the anonymity of authors. The accounts and bullying behaviours described are wide ranging, thought-provoking but overall sad and heart-wrenching. The passion and commitment of these midwives and their love for the art and science of midwifery and the women that they care for are clear. Many reading these accounts, will empathise with the midwives, understanding how they feel as they may have been bullied themselves or will have seen or heard their colleagues being bullied. Ultimately, bullying within midwifery exists in a permissive toxic culture which results in midwives being harmed and many leaving their job, the profession and even the country to get away from the bully. Tragically, in some cases, being bullied, leads to self-harm and contemplation of or actual suicide.

The following accounts have been read, reread and thematically analysed, leading to the development of 6 main themes and 24 subthemes. All the themes relate to midwives leaving or thinking about leaving their job or profession Some of the accounts cross over themes but in order to keep the accounts as they were told, they are located under the main theme where it is thought that there is a best fit. ***The quote/s which fits with the main themes in each of the midwives' accounts is in bolded text.***

However, reading the full account, provides insight into the awful reality of bullying for the midwives and the women they care for.

Table 1 displays the 6 main themes and the 24 subthemes identified within the midwives and Midwife Support Worker (MSW) accounts. The overarching theme is that of bullying behaviours which led to working conditions that were unacceptable and negatively impacting on the midwives- the triggers for leaving (or in a small number of cases staying as they felt they had no choice) may be different but these midwives were bullied, and/or had witnessed bullying of their colleagues and women who were accessing maternity services.

Table 1: Themes and subthemes identified within the accounts

THEMES	SUB THEMES
A. Leave their job and move to another midwifery job to get away from the bully/bullying	Bullying by clique of managers and work life balance
	Negative impact on health and well-being and bystander effect
	Lack of managerial support; failure to tackle bullying by management/ workplace Union
	Could not question the narrative and seeing women bullied into decisions about their care
	Poor working conditions including lack of recognition of skills and reasonable adjustments
	Managers bullied for supporting staff concerns about working conditions
	Unrealistic expectations-Continuity of Care provision/on-call requirements

THEMES	SUB THEMES
B. Leave their midwifery job in UK	Lack of individualism- being expected to conform
C. Thinking of leaving	Impact on health and well-being
	Blame Culture
D. Leave midwifery and move to another role in or outside of healthcare	Negativity and lack of positive feedback
	Grieve for no longer being a midwife
E. Left Midwifery	Bullied into unnecessary intervention
	Working conditions, impacting on standard of care
	Targeted with unfounded allegations
	Bullied by known bully
	Bullied as a midwife and received poor care as woman
	Negative impact on health and well-being
F. Staying as need to work	Persistent bullying that is not addressed
	Bully seems untouchable
	Bullying in academic settings
	Preferential treatment and not being listened to
	Working conditions and racism
	Feeling suicidal

A. Leave their Job and Moving to another Midwifery Role to get away from the Bully

Bullying by Clique of Managers and Work Life Balance

Bullying from managers and the challenge of reaching an acceptable work/life balance, has led this midwife to re-evaluate and move to a new role within midwifery.

"Bullying, shift patterns, no work-life balance, burnout. ***Working in abortion care now and can honestly say it's the happiest I've been since I started my training. I trained and worked at a Trust where bullying was endemic. Delivery suite was ruled by a core group of Band 7s who could make or break the midwives. I saw midwives of 20+ years reduced to tears by their nastiness, midwives leave or be driven out sick due to bullying. I approached the chief exec as a whistle blower, some action was taken and two of the band 7s encouraged to take early retirement to prevent further investigation into the bullying claims.*** *One was given 'gardening leave' but returned after a few months because the 40+ reports of bullying weren't sufficient evidence. The matron at the time accessed my personal health record but was allowed to keep her position! These women have now all retired and the matron finally downgraded to a band 6 midwife but the damage they caused was simply horrific and sadly they've left their legacy behind with a new core band of bullying band 7s and a truly toxic work environment. I now work at another Trust where bullying isn't an issue and the support amongst colleagues is phenomenal.* ***Sadly, the management is poor.*** *We have steamrolled ahead with CoC despite not having the staff numbers to accommodate it.* ***Heaven forbid you say anything negative about CoC though, even our head obstetrician was silenced by the actions of the CoC lead. Every shift is short staffed, the unit is far from safe. Concerns have been raised at the highest level outside of maternity, but even their attitude is dismissive now. Nobody is listening. But hey, we're trailblazers for CoC and that's all that matters right?"***

Negative Impact on Health and Well-Being and Bystander Effect

Midwives who were bullied and left, subsequently spent a lot of time rebuilding their confidence and health and well-being, with some not feeling able to work for a while with the impact spreading into personal and family life. There are also accounts of midwives who have considered suicide. The Bystander effect is also highlighted here with those who are bullied not understanding why colleagues don't try to help.

"I have had a similar experience in the past at a previous Trust and was bullied out. Didn't work for a while then went to another Trust where I have felt welcomed, appreciated and supported. It's a totally different experience. It took me a long time to rebuild my confidence and I'm still working on that but it does get easier."

"I have been a midwife for many years and given it my life and soul. I remain full of passion, dedication and love for everything that is midwifery and the NHS. *I have watched and supported colleagues who have experienced bullying over the years and thought it would never happen to me but I was wrong.* ***A few years ago I had the best job I had ever had and successfully carried it out but was bullied so badly first by my manager then by the wider management team (on her recommendation). I considered ending my life, not once but twice and nobody knew until recently which was very difficult for them to hear and understand.*** *I can't actually talk about what happened because I have now worked through the trauma in more ways than one and it could damage the repair but the* ***sequence of events were extraordinary and quite honestly unbelievably inhumane.*** *I do hope to share some of the things I learnt one day to help others either in writing or conference but I still live in fear so this won't be in the near future.* ***What happened to me was so damaging that it affected me as both as a person and almost ruined both my professional and personal life, on reflection it even inadvertently affected my next job. The detrimental effect was phenomenal,*** *but I am so grateful that now I have turned the corner, although, not without a lot of work on myself. On reading the accounts of my fellow colleagues' experiences I no longer feel alone, which I find both extremely sad but reassuring because there is always a self-blame attached to bullying and that is what perpetrators are particularly good at. I never really felt validated in the way I was feeling but questioned what it was I had done to deserve it, now I see it as why did they think it was ok to treat me in that way?* ***One of my biggest concerns is not always the person who bullies but how shameful it is when others notice but do nothing, I will never understand this.***

I really don't know if there is anything that can be done but I sincerely hope that by giving people a voice will help commence the healing and bring us all together. I also hope that anyone in this group who has been a bully to others will recognise themselves and the effect their actions have then ask for support to help them improve their behaviour or situation."

This midwife recounts how challenging the Head of Midwifery (HOM) led to threats about losing her job, leading to her needing medication and having to change jobs.

"Even us strong midwives of over many years in senior positions get bullied. *I have been reading accounts on a daily basis and they are heart breaking.* ***I have been a midwife for many years and given it everything I have.*** *I was rotational for many years, then a ward manager and then a specialist midwife. A few years ago, I loved my job but then acted up for a senior member of staff who was off sick for 9 months. I was told by the HOM that 'the difference you make is palpable' but I was not afraid to challenge my HOM in a professional way. An interview for a permanent post came up and I was unsuccessful. (Not my best I admit).* ***I returned to my original specialist midwife post and was told twice in front of my manager, by the HOM that 'my job was on the line' if we did not achieve the accreditation expected. She was dismissive and did not engage with me except to criticise. Her dismissive management style (my way or no way) plus the team she brought in who were exactly the same, resulted with me on antidepressants and feeling like I needed to leave. It took 18 months for the behaviours to finally hit me.*** *My stomach would churn as I approached the building. What happened to me felt so damaging and I thank God for my family, friends and colleagues who got me through it.* ***I detest bullying in any way and it needs stamping out. On a positive note, I now have a positive and supportive HOM and Deputy HOM and love my job again."***

Lack of Managerial Support; Failure to Tackle Bullying by Management/Union

This midwife recounts a lack of support and acceptance by management/workplace Union that some midwives are bullies. Her experiences have had a long-term impact on her health and well-being.

"I have been qualified since xxxx, I worked at the Trust I trained at initially, really enjoyed it and felt like a valued member of the team. Two years later, I was over the moon to be successful at getting a core job on delivery suite and felt like I'd found my work home. Shortly after I started my core job one of the band 7 delivery suite midwives ***stopped me in the corridor mid shift to tell me that she didn't think I was good enough for core and I shouldn't have got the job. I was speechless.*** *The following day I received an email from another band 6 to tell me that the same band 7 had asked her to email me on her behalf to inform me that the student who was working with me would no longer be my student. I arranged an urgent meeting*

with the manager, she said that she would discuss this with the band 7. Nothing further was done.

In March of this year the same band 7 asked me to meet with her in one of the offices on the unit. I agreed, a little annoyed that this took me from my clinical duties but hoped it would be a short chat and that I could continue with my work. She then proceeded to tell me that she had concerns about me and that I still wasn't good enough to be working in the unit and that she had decided that she was going to speak to HR to have me removed. ***She then started asking about my mental health and because I had received help from the staff support team due to my own previous experiences in the theatres (I almost died following a surgical error [detail removed to anonymise]) that it was another reason why I wasn't suitable. I couldn't believe that this woman, was putting me down again and using my mental health as a tool against me.*** *I honestly couldn't believe what I was hearing. This happened on the eve of some annual leave I had so I spent that week off in a state of anxiety and paranoia.*

I returned to work the following week and confided in a senior midwife who said she would support my temporary move to another area whilst this was sorted out. I also informed her that I'd started applying for other jobs as I no longer felt safe in the Trust. I had a meeting with the matron, ***I told her I felt bullied yet again by this one band 7, she calmly said "maybe she will retire"!!! I then informed her that I was considering leaving because of this, again, she calmly said "ok, that's fine" and I knew I was never going to feel like I belonged there again.***

I spoke to the union rep midwife, was told I needed to arrange a mediation meeting with my bully. I knew I couldn't put myself through that, and that's what I said. They said there was nothing else they could offer me in terms of support. I spoke to a freedom to speak to guardian, she sent me the bullying policy and that was that.

I arranged a meeting with someone in HR, they sent my concerns back to the HOM who emailed me promptly as I had raised safeguarding concerns not only for staff but for the women we were providing care for. ***I'd left the Trust at this point but our emails went back and forth for a few weeks before she informed me that she had spoken with the matron and they had plans for how they were going to improve the Trust, and she hoped I was well.***

I couldn't believe it. My concerns feel ignored. I feel like I didn't matter and I wasn't a valued member of that team. *That this one individual had done the Trust a favour by getting rid of me.*

I am now working in a different Trust *and I'm overwhelmed by how lovely and supportive everyone is. I've got a long way to go until my workplace anxiety and* *confidence changes but* ***I feel like I've made the right move.*** *I've recently been diagnosed with xx and this experience has definitely played a part in this. When I initially went to my GP about my health concerns, he didn't want to put the referral in as he knew how I was being treated at work and was concerned that it would make my working conditions much worse. I'm glad I stuck up for myself and stood my ground. I'm now able to access the help I need."*

"Until xx this ***year, I was an NHS Nurse and Midwife. I worked and loved my role for 20 years but after a horrific year of watching myself and my colleagues suffering the most appalling bullying I left.*** *I am currently still receiving support for the trauma but I am now working for an employer that values me and pays me well. What most concerned me about this incident is that despite numerous reports of bullying and harassment and unsafe staffing to even the Chief Executive; nothing was done."*

This midwife describes being exposed to bullying behaviour since being a student midwife and as a midwife learning how to cope with the bullying and getting involved in working with a Union in order to help others and change the bullying culture. However, following a promotion, bullying behaviour escalated from a clique of midwives which eventually had a detrimental impact on her health and well-being.

"My experience of bullying started when I was a student midwife. On my first day as a student my mentor said 'oh god not another student' and during my placement ignored me whenever I spoke. She always walked a few paces in front of me when we were on community visits. ***I'd waited 13 years to realise my dream to become a midwife, I wasn't going to let this stop me now. The team told me not to let her bother me, she was often like this.*** *In labour ward, however, the bullying was worse, mostly it was the Band 7 Charge midwives who seemed to enjoy putting students down (one in particular was bad). But there were other midwives who were undermining and patronising too.* ***They didn't just pick on students, they did it to any midwives who weren't in their clique. I reached out to the Union for support to deal with this as a student and they told me there had been institutional bullying in the maternity Trust I was placed on, for nearly 2 decades and they were working with HR to create Dignity at Work policies****. They encouraged me to get involved, so I did.*

(Piece of text removed to maintain anonymity)

"Staff confided in me when they had any health and safety concerns (including bullying) and I helped them report it. I got on well with colleagues in the 3-4 years I was a qualified midwife and learned how to navigate the bullying. The real problem for me however started when I was promoted to a band 7 post in xxx. From my first day I felt shocked and a feeling of fear came over me when, on my first day as a Band 7, one of my labour ward, Band 7 colleagues blanked me. There was no congratulations in my new role. We'd always been on talking terms before so I was surprised. Another took me into her office on day 2, and told me I shouldn't have been promoted as I hadn't been qualified long enough and she said that she and the Band 7 senior charge midwives in labour ward wouldn't be helping me. *I reported this to my manager but my band 7 colleague denied she'd said this. The team I managed in the birth unit then started to report incidences where transfers were being blocked or women unnecessarily delayed between the birth unit and labour ward when they needed labour ward care. There were reports that some registrars had declined to sign prescription Kardex when midwives asked them, and one B7 mentioned on several occasions the B7 labour ward staff would no longer be responding to emergency buzzers anymore if they went off in the birth unit. The B7s began taking staff from the birth unit leaving me to staff the unit alone. The reasons were not reasonable ones, but they overruled me at every turn.* ***They gave me the silent treatment, belittled me at huddles and referred to the birth unit team at B7 meetings as 'duff', and made allegations that the birth unit team were dangerous, unsafe practitioners but declined to give details when I offered to look into this.*** *(I did check notes however and found care to be safe and appropriate). They told me I'd need to earn the respect of the B7s, that it didn't matter I'd been a B6 colleague before.*

I continued to report these communications to my line manager and she said she saw what they were doing and that she was dealing with it. She told me she had been bullied by some of them as a student and as a midwife too and that she had my back. Other senior managers took me aside to ask how I was coping. They each had their own stories and the common theme was that the labour ward B7s were a 'strong bunch, look after yourself and know how they operate, it's been like this for decades, they rule the roost, they're bullies.' *I raised this with the HOM and she said she'd look into it, I said if she didn't do something I'd raise this with the NMC as I was concerned about the safety of women and babies. The team of midwives in the birth unit began to pass onto me stories of their experiences of being bullied and undermined by Labour ward B7s when I was off shift. The HOM told me she spoke to the B7s and told them to stop saying the things they were, to stop closing the birth unit overnight and taking the birth unit staff to labour ward without reporting/escalating the reasons for this.* ***But the next***

day one of the B7s told me they didn't care what Management said, they'll do what they want anyway as there's more of them than me. It was horrendous. I started to feel really anxious going to work but determined they wouldn't get me down.

My line manager continued to offer support and said she was dealing with it and that their manager would be performance managing them. She told me I was doing a great job, to hang in there as it would get better. The birth unit team started to file Datix about the behaviours and resulting impact on women and babies to help give management evidence of the bullying. ***But the situation got worse. My manager, who had said all along she supported me and was dealing with the behaviour through the proper channels, let slip she hadn't done anything and that no one was being performance managed. I expressed my shock. She then called me into an unscheduled meeting the next day and said all the B7s wanted to complain about me.*** *None of the allegations they made were founded and I showed my manager evidence of this. She said she didn't think it could be all of them and not me.* ***I realised then they were all mob bullying me. I've never felt so terrified in my life.*** *I reached out to the Union.* ***The Union's position was an eye opener. They said that because there were several instead of 7 x Band 7s in labour ward and just me in the birth unit my chances of successfully doing anything about this were slim.*** *They said they see it all the time that birth unit teams are frequently undermined by labour ward B7s and that if I was to action the dignity at work policy it would be traumatic for me, it would affect my mental health, and the B7s would likely lie about me; and because there's more of them, they'll win. They said the HOM would likely rule that my being in post destabilises the service and makes care of women and babies unsafe. I was completely gobsmacked and devastated. A career I'd waited for so long to do, a promotion I'd worked extremely hard for ... gone in that moment.* ***I couldn't go back and realised I'd nowhere and no one to turn to. I asked the Union what they would do about the bullying culture in labour ward as they knew it was decades old.*** *I had kept a file of my situation, emails from B7s and medical staff, text messages, where bullying was evident, but they didn't want to see it. What they agreed to do was a 1 hour non-mandatory workshop for staff on bullying. I couldn't believe it.*

On the Union's advice ***I took time off sick to give me time to recover and find another job. I felt very lucky to gain employment as xxx, but that hasn't been without its challenges either.*** *Firstly, we had a bully in the team who gave me and another member of staff the silent treatment at work for about 8 weeks and remained frosty with me until she retired. This was because she shouted at a student and I asked her not to do that. As a practice education lecturer in my educator role, I now support students who experience challenges in the placement* *areas and there's several complaints about bullying I have had and am currently dealing with, mostly B7 labour ward charge midwives, including in the area I've referred to here.* ***I also see bullying behaviours in some students towards students and towards lecturing staff.*** *I still miss clinical practice, working with women and babies was my greatest joy, but it turned to horror. My job became untenable for myself as a midwife in the same way it has done for hundreds of other midwives - I have women centred values centred on building relationships on mutual respect, human regard, effective communication and professionalism. Something I find to be lacking among many members of staff I've worked with. Most are derogatory about women and if you don't operate at this level you'll never fully be accepted as one of the team, you'll be ostracised and the service will spit you out.*

*Most midwives fear losing their career and income (understandably) if they speak up therefore, they succumb to these behaviours in order to survive. It's heart-breaking and I'm still grieving nearly 5 years on. A colleague of mine summed it up well. 'The problem with ******** is that she's all about the women and the staff don't like that'. The government need to have change agents and leadership experts go into the maternity service en masse. I believe it could be sorted if they had good courageous leaders in there to tackle it.* ***At the moment sending hundreds of students into this mess is next to pointless, so many are confused, anxious and traumatised and as we know, so many will leave.*** *I'd relish the opportunity to lead* change, with the right backing."

Could not Question the Narrative and Seeing Women Bullied into Decisions about their Care

These midwives felt that they could not ask questions and were seeing women bullied into decisions about their care, and eventually left the NHS.

"Ok. ***Why I'm no longer an NHS midwife.*** *Despite the rhetoric of 'Evidence Based Medicine', the evidence regarding anything to do with natural (not normal, people's version of normal has become quite concerning), is almost always ignored, due to fear of litigation. Women feel bullied into investigations, vaccines, internals, etc. They enter the birthing machine and get spat out the other end often with PTSD. Not surprising given that a huge proportion of midwives themselves too, experience off the scale trauma. I was bullied from the first day of my first ever placement, by a midwife, who of course is now, 24 years later, very high up in Management of the Trust she still remains in. I remember being sick in the car park every morning such was my fear. I was moved to another hospital as I was deemed to be the problem, daring to suggest that bullying had occurred.*

*Fortunately, at my next hospital, I remained until qualifying (on labour ward at least), with a beautiful soul and my faith was slightly restored. Then, you qualify (1999), and I galloped around the globe gathering as much experience as I could muster, from the xx to xx. Then back to the UK. The amalgamations of smaller trusts, to bigger trusts, the closing of almost all birth centres (to then at best be replaced by birth centres next door to labour wards, run by high-risk midwives who have a fast diminishing idea of what natural birth dare to look like, my last visit to one, being told the birth ejection reflex was a myth of an imaginative mind by the band 7 co-ordinator, but I digress)! **Bullying is endemic throughout most Trusts I have been in. The insidious ways they find to bully you. Dare to question the narrative, by God your life is hell. My last NHS xx job, came to an abrupt end when I questioned on a study day our vaccine information leaflet for whooping cough.** The leaflet discussed whooping cough only and why the vaccine was important. It gave zero information that the vaccine was a 3 in 1 (at that time), including whooping cough. I asked if this was informed consent? This clearly was one step too far in my questioning mind, was quickly labelled an 'anti vaxer' (not sure where that bomb came from), and within a week I got a P45 from the Trust as I hadn't submitted a shift in 3 months (I had, and I'd been on study days with them). That was my last day in an NHS building in a midwife capacity. So now my Master's Degree in Midwifery and all these 24 years of experience is locked in my head with nowhere to go.*

I miss women immensely** (but stay registered through other private work), but I don't miss providing substandard care, surrounded by substandard humans dressed in uniforms calling themselves midwives. I'm back to nursing, which is hugely unfortunate. **I'm a good nurse, but I was a much, much better midwife."

The repercussions for the next midwife of supporting women in their choices had far-reaching consequences on her health and well-being, including feeling suicidal, leading to changing jobs and leaving the NHS.

"I am a registered midwife, no longer working in the NHS.** I qualified in 2007 and loved my job with all my heart. I was good at it too. During my career I worked in intrapartum care on a consultant led delivery suite in an inner-city hospital with a bad management reputation. There was a bullying culture and a blame culture which I tried to steer clear of. **But I was a tall poppy. I couldn't help but speak for the women, to help them achieve better births, to not tolerate bad practices and to try to introduce best practice. It was hard, hard work but my colleagues on the shop floor were supportive- it was management who were not.

I was first bullied early in my career by my team leader who picked on me, pulled my notes for minor errors and made it clear she didn't like me.

In xxxx, I was involved in an incident where I was unfairly and unjustly treated by the midwifery management structure (not just my opinion but that of many colleagues, consultant obstetricians and my union rep). ***As soon as I tried to discuss my case, management shut me down, took me out of clinical practice and the nightmare began as I fought to clear my name and save my career*** *(I had just returned from a year out doing an MSc). After a torturous YEAR I did but was so disgusted with my treatment and lack of support I left that Trust to go elsewhere.*

However, the damage was done. ***My physical and mental health were so damaged by the process that I could no longer cope. I had PTSD from the bullying and the incident, had started smoking again (I had quit 3 years previously) and was self-medicating with alcohol on a regular basis and had even contemplated suicide.*** *I couldn't sleep well, had recurrent nightmares and my blood pressure needed urgent attention (200/120!). I had to leave clinical midwifery before it killed me.*

Since leaving I have recovered, but I am still in contact with midwife friends from this Trust who tell me it's worse than ever, *midwives being told* ***it's either the management's way or they can leave- and many do, when all they want are reasonable working conditions and flexible working as they have children.*** *I have been forwarded emails which are bullying and threatening staff with repercussions if they do not comply to unreasonable demands from them. It's tragic that experienced midwives are just dispensable in a climate where we are desperate for staff, and then replaced with terrified newly qualified midwives who, let's face it, will eventually leave in the same way, after the same humiliating and inhumane treatment I have received myself and witnessed first-hand doled out to others.*

So, what's the answer you may ask? Well, I don't know, but I have midwife friends throughout the country and a dominant theme is the management culture. We all talk about the wrong people getting into positions of power- midwives who didn't enjoy caring for women and families usually. ***Current management choose the next managers (replicas of themselves) and groom them ready to take their positions. It's a perpetuating cycle of badness. Management needs a complete overhaul. It needs people with hearts at its heart not people who don't care, are unable to think outside the box and seem dead behind the eyes.***

It's too late for me which is such a shame as I had so much more to give to my clinical midwifery career, but the thought of subjecting myself to that again fills me with terror. It's not too late for others though, the future midwives who need to feel valued, supported and nurtured. Good midwives give so much great care, but they need caring for themselves to do this, not abusing.

I say I've recovered, and I have- a lot- but I cried throughout writing this and that is wrong. ***Someone needs to stop people feeling like me and other midwives do, all we wanted was to go to work and do a good job."***

Poor Working Conditions, including Lack of Recognition of Skills and Reasonable Adjustments

These midwives recount how they felt undervalued, had poor working conditions, were bullied, felt unable to do anything about it, to the point that they couldn't work in midwifery anymore.

"I left midwifery last year after 16 years. It was a mixture of feeling my skills were unrecognised, being bullied for the first time in my life, and realising that absolutely nothing would be done about it, and the way we were treated during Covid, being told we were not allowed to wear PPE was a particular low point. *I am still registered but have almost completed my health visiting training. The difference in the care and compassion I have been shown is marked. I feel very sad that I have left a team that I loved but the on-calls were ridiculous, being expected to do 12.5 hours on call after working a 7.5 day, being called to any part of the county to staff the MLUs or home births and of course into delivery suite when busy. I can't believe I lasted as long as I did. It's a shame because I know I am a good and passionate midwife who loved having students and providing women centred care. I am just not prepared to work like that anymore."*

"I left midwifery last year. As a mature student I had had to sacrifice a lot to consider going back to full time education, putting off buying a house, having children etc. etc. but it was my passion so I qualified in xxxx. During the training itself I had encountered and been witness to horrific bullying behaviour however I had my rose-tinted glasses on and just thought 'it's going to be OK now I'm qualified, *I've worked so hard to get here and I am not throwing my 3 years of training away to go back to my old job'.. I thought a new Trust was the answer, because other trusts can 'surely be nicer' so off I went from a busy maternity unit near London to a much smaller "calmer" hospital in the East of England. I have to say my hope for things to be completely different were somewhat the opposite.* ***I had no proper induction, no one showed me where theatres were if I had a patient who needed to be taken there, no one showed me round the birthing rooms or even orientated me to the toilets or drug cupboard... I was given the constant smirk and eye roll 'oh YOU are the new community midwife; we'll see how long you last' whilst giggling to one another about me.*** *I was* *somewhat initially relieved to go out to community and be away from it. I loved my community job and would have stayed there for the rest of my days if I was allowed to do exactly that.   community! It was manic and busy and we constantly had lovely students come out on placement from working on labour ward shocked at how busy we were because the hospital midwives had told them how we were lazy and drink tea all day... oh, the irony!*

After working all day, we would be called out often on the way back to our homes after a day without lunch or drinks and be asked to go straight to help on labour ward. *Now we were supposed to only work for 4 hours then be allowed to go home. that was the rule and my manager had clearly instructed me to warn them after 3.5 hrs that I would be going when we hit 4 hours as my team needed me the next day to help cover clinics and visits etc. .. As in community we are supposed to be 'low risk', we are supposed to reflect that whilst going in the hospital, however I would often rock up to be allocated the patient on a sliding scale or the pre-eclamptic woman. ..they would all be gathered round me in the office when I asked why I couldn't have the low risk multiple that was making her way in .... 'because we have been working all night and it's time for the community to start using some brain cells, what's the matter you can't cope' all whilst side glancing at one another and smirking. Quite frankly no I couldn't. . as a community midwife I hadn't looked after a woman on a sliding scale since I was a student. ...so, it wasn't fair on myself or the woman and actually was quite unsafe, they should have been looking after the woman as high risk was their 'bread and butter' so to speak. I muddled my way through feeling unworthy, unconfident and ganged up on. I went back to the office to update my board whilst they were all their eating cake.... why, oh why had I been called in... to be made an example of?!* ***After 3.5 hrs I went to the co-ordinator who was sat around her bullying gang, pre-warned her that we were approaching 4 hours and I would be going so who could I hand over to? 'You are supposed to be a midwife, I don't know if you know but that is supposed to mean "with woman" and it says a lot about you as a person if you are happy to leave your woman in her hour of need. ..there isn't anyone to hand over to we are all busy can't you see that. ..no I guess you can't because you community midwives aren't the most observant people are you?' I said I felt unsafe and was ignored, I said I needed to go and was ignored.***

Should I just leave but then would I get in trouble for not handing over to someone and my patient would be the one to suffer, so no I stayed under duress whilst they cackled the night away in their office taking night shift selfies to upload to Facebook and Tik Tok. I ended up leaving when the day staff came on shift. I had had no lunch, no dinner and barely anything to drink and my clinic started in 2 hours with no one to cover it. I left the hospital but felt like I could barely keep my eyes open so pulled over in a lay-by and slept then drove straight to my clinic. ***I escalated it to the band 8 manager and spoke of the Tik Tok and social media evidence proving they weren't rushed off their feet as they made out. ...she said 'you are being a bit silly aren't you. the hospital staff have been through horrific things during covid and if they want to do that to boost morale then so be it'... broken I was right there in that moment. the luxury of having time to take selfies. the fact that the community staff had been made to go into home to carry out home visits or home births without any PPE at the start of covid because the little PPE there was, prioritised for the hospital staff.*** *The team had been dropping like flies testing positive one after another, and yet this is our management and our form of 'support' whilst she had laid in her comfy bed all night long whilst I had not stopped. Where is the fairness in that?! I started to build anxiety and a bit of PTSD towards going in there so I took myself off the PDM to gain some support... well, I wish I hadn't bothered...I was given a woman that needed to be go for a crash section. still at this point I did not know where theatres were or anything despite asking time and time again. I told the PDM that I felt like running away, I felt unsafe, didn't know where anything was etc...****She put her hand up to my face and said 'STOP ..if you want to run away, do it but there will be significant repercussions for you. ...you are clearly not cut out to be a midwife and if you haven't got it in you then I can't miracle it to put it in you. You are clearly out of your depth and need to look at other jobs. supermarkets have lots of vacancies you know'.***

That was it. ..totally crushed, any ounce of confidence I had in me had been eliminated in that moment. She was supposed to be the form of support. . instead she was like the others - corrupt and a bully to the core. *Maybe I wasn't cut out for this. ..but I had come from working on a busy obstetric unit completing my preceptorship and working in theatres and was a confident midwife. This place had broken me. Since then, a midwife has gone to the papers reporting bullying about this unit. Nothing has been done the Head of Midwifery says it isn't up for discussion and will not address it. The CQC have found poor management and leadership and the hospital's answer was to employ more managers who, like the existing managers, stay in their offices when the staffing is dangerously short and patient care is compromised alongside practitioners' well-being of not having breaks etc.* ***I left and feel ashamed and upset that they won and ruined my dream career but my dream career is changing rapidly and the bullying ethos is just worsening and is being continuously swept under the carpet. Management need to be held accountable. Bullying cliques need to be broken up and practitioners need to feel safe and supported in carrying out their role."***

"For the majority of my 10 years I think I was extremely lucky after reading so many awful stories. I have worked with so many amazing and supportive midwives. However, I have experienced bullying within this and this is one example... On a busy labour ward night shift I was continually asked to care for an excessive number of women. The unit was busy and staffing was short. ***I repeatedly refused to take on more work informing the coordinator it was not safe and I wanted to keep my [NMC] PIN number. I asked her to call the manager on call and the SoM {Supervisor of Midwives]. Eventually I caved after realising one of the women she wanted me to take over had a midwife with her who was supposed to have finished her 12 hour shift 2 hours previously. It was a horrible shift but thankfully nothing bad happened. No supervisor came to the unit the whole night. I informed the coordinator the following morning I was going to fill out an incident report before I left due to unsafe staffing levels. She said that was fine. I spoke to the SoM the following day- she had had no phone call overnight and I felt so let down.***

Following submission of my incident report the coordinator no longer spoke to me on shift unless absolutely necessary. She ignored me in corridors and rooms, ensuring no eye contact or recognition of me being there. She referred to me by name only if she had a direct question or for allocation. I could not go to her for support on shift. This went on for months. I have no doubt to the pressures she was under but that is not an excuse to treat a colleague like they no longer matter. ***It was a time of bullying upper management in the hospital where you would not dare eat a biscuit or have a drink on shift in case you were "caught"*** *(text removed to protect anonymity). After reading so many heart-breaking student accounts on FB, I am certainly apprehensive of what I might find out about local Trusts, but know without the info we can't help."*

This account is from a midwife with a disability whose reasonable adjustments were not accommodated.

"The reality we all live is horrific & I'm sure if the women knew how we are being forced to work they would be against it. Anonymously - ***I'd like to know just how many midwives there are who have long term health conditions/disabilities or even short-term health issues who have been forced to leave, bullied, harassed & not been given reasonable adjustments which are more than reasonable and are legally allowed to support their health/well-being at work which in turn creates better safety, efficiency & productivity for this particular group of midwives?*** *Have the unions managed to fight for you under the equality act & won or have you simply given up? Has HR been supportive if you have taken if further?*

There's no real discussion etc about midwives with disabilities whether that be mental health, physical, visible or invisible and I feel there are more out there than is realised but as we are expected to be robots and fulfil 'service needs' we are frightened to declare it & being forced to continue as we are or give up because midwifery has no place for staff with health issues *God forbid staff's health is becoming more complex as well as the patients & god forbid we actually care about our staff as well as the patients!"*

Managers Bullied for Supporting Staff Concerns about Working Conditions

Managers also found that they were subjected to bullying also, including when they felt that they were supporting their staff.

"I just wanted to emphasise that Managers who don't toe the line but try and fight for their staff are victimised and bullied out of the service too. I still have lots of regrets about leaving and guilt that I couldn't have stayed to support my work family but the situation was impossible. *Things at that Trust have got even worse and many more good midwives and managers have left, to be replaced by Band 5s. This is deeply unfair to those NQM who are not getting the support they deserve.*

I still find myself even now supporting midwives from my previous Trust who contact me privately for advice.

The whole management team has now been replaced and yet no one questions why that is. ***Easier to sweep under the carpet."***

Unrealistic Expectations of Continuity of Care Provision/On-Call Requirements

This midwife left her job as she was working in unsustainable work rotas and then were bullied for questioning this.

"I left a job last year after working in a CoC team for 3 years. It was soul destroying, expected to work 12.5 hours if called in after working a 7.5 hour shift. We were on call 2 times a week. I was a team leader and saw many staff burn out. We were 6FTE and in my time there we went through 15 FTE and there was 19 episodes of long term sickness. I tried speaking up to maternity SLT (Senior Leadership Team) and was branded a troublemaker and bullied out of the Trust. I've given midwifery one last try at a new Trust where I'm happy, but if CoC was ever introduced to my team I'd leave midwifery. Whilst I'm happy where I am,

I feel privileged, I'm in a specialist team and don't do on calls. The community midwives are regularly called in, despite the policy saying they can only work 5 hours this rarely happens. It's soul destroying."

B. Leave their Midwifery Job in UK

Lack of Individualism

This midwife felt that they could not express their individuality and also felt that practice was unsafe and underpaid.

"Work felt like a prison- ***no creative expression, must all look the same,*** *can't be neurodivergent, must play by rules...* ***must accept all the terrible conditions and not complain.*** *I'm in midwifery still but left the UK because it was unsafe and underpaid... plus toxic work culture- does that count?"*

C. Thinking of Leaving

Impact on health and well-being

These midwives are thinking about leaving due to the cumulative effect of bullying behaviours that they have been exposed to. The negative impact on their health is clear but they can't leave for personal reasons.

"I am thinking about leaving, I have had enough and don't want to go to an early grave. Just figuring out where to go with a xx yr. old."

"In fact this came up in my memories of 2 years ago today. 'Everybody is all "yay Friday!" but I'm working my 4th of 7 weekends in a row. Who needs a social life and to see their family anyway?' It was about 6 weeks after this that I left a Friday night shift at 3am ***(despite being told to "pull myself together" by a shift lead) and was signed off for over a month by my GP."***

"I trained to be a midwife xx years ago and truly loved it, *from the moment I started. All of it, dipping urine, palpating and finally working out what I was feeling. Feeling that amazing rush when a woman and I locked eyes and we traversed a beautiful journey together. I often said 'I can't believe they'll actually pay me to do this!'* ***I loved it so much I'd have happily done it for free.*** *In the beginning of my third year I fell out with one of our cohort, it was a minor thing and I thought we'd work it out,* ***she was a popular person with the 'in crowd' and the bullying culture at our Trust was rife. Once I fell out with her my life changed very quickly there. Midwives refused to work with me, I was ignored through whole night shifts, spending my breaks in the toilet or the closed antenatal clinic which was more bearable than being in a staffroom and ignored. Other students had left the course because of the brutal bullying there and it was just accepted. Some were advised to go out drinking with them to 'get in with them', the in- group was pretty impenetrable.***

A senior midwife worked with me for a whole shift and I was dreading it, she had a fierce reputation for being a hard and nasty person. I got through the shift with her and learnt a lot, I'd felt a bit useless at times but she'd explained that she needed to be short with me because of lack of time to get messages across. I felt that maybe I had misjudged her and that she was professional above being cruel. We sat in the busy staffroom afterwards and she tried to convince me that the baby we had delivered had a rare condition, she fetched a neonatal text book and pretended to read from it. In the room were other midwives and a couple of doctors, she suggested that I 'write my next essay on it'. ***It was only on my way home that it dawned on me that she was winding me up and just wanting to make me look stupid in front of the other people in the room.***

By the end of the course, whenever I spoke in class the back 2 rows in the classroom would whisper and take the mick out of me, I was so close to leaving but I couldn't because I'd invested too much. By the end I was having panic attacks and was on antidepressants. *I had spoken to another senior midwife for advice and support, she told the other midwife and no support was offered to me as I wasn't prepared to make an official complaint. I finished the course, took some time off, I needed a break, did some voluntary work and built my confidence back up. A year later I went for a job interview there, I was given the first interview of the day, left in a corridor for almost an hour while one of them (the midwife with the textbook) went to go and get some breakfast. When they finally interviewed me, she intimidated me throughout the interview saying repeatedly 'sorry you've got to talk to me now' every time she was asking the interview questions. The other NQM's who had been interviewed had been offered jobs by 5 o'clock that evening,*

I hadn't heard anything by 7pm. After calling the SMWs office a couple of times, she called me and told me they wouldn't be offering me the job because they didn't feel I was safe to practise.

I had 3 years off work in total and had to have counselling before I did a return to practice and got a job in different Trust. *There were many other small incidences that happened but they seem so insignificant singularly. They all culminated in totally wrecking my confidence and mental health. I practised happily (and safely!) for 6 years in the other Trust and returned to my initial Trust a few years ago. It hasn't really changed there,* ***a few of the same nasty women are still there, I've been shouted at in a corridor in front of other members of staff (to their utter disbelief) and had my practice questioned, luckily, I'm meticulous and so far, a couple of attempts to discredit me have been unsuccessful.***

In the last 5 months, my daughter was pregnant after many years of sad losses. She was going to have her baby in our Trust and I was able to ask friends to care for her. ***When it came time to have her baby, this midwife had decided that, because of COVID, I wouldn't be able to be at the birth as well as her partner, she met with the midwifery managers to ensure that I wouldn't be able to be there. Before my daughter and after, other staff members have been able to support family members in addition to the 1 birth partner, I am the only person that such effort was made to ensure I wouldn't be breaking this 'important COVID guideline'****. There's a lot more to this story obviously, insinuating that I was a safeguarding risk, my swipe card not working in the 2 weeks that I was off.* ***The most important thing is that my daughter and I weren't able to share such an important moment.*** *One of the basic perks of being a midwife is being able to provide that support to the ones you love as well as treating strangers with the same care that you would your daughter.* ***I have been looking for jobs outside of midwifery now, along with some huge professional grievances, I just can't stay there any longer.*** *I'm considering taking a grievance out on this midwife but in my heart, I know there's no point,* ***I just need to leave.*** *At core, I still think it's the most beautiful job in the world but our Trust is so badly managed, (we've had 35 resignations since April) I cannot keep doing this to myself.* ***I'm back on antidepressants and have been having panic attacks again, this time it feels so much more vindictive and personal and I just can't stay in a place that values people so little."***

"I wanted to tell my story (anonymously) about my difficulties during my 15 year midwifery career. ***I really wish I could be more positive and uplifting but at the moment I'm on leave long term with mental health problems and at a real crossroads as to how I can continue in the profession that I have worked so hard***

and sacrificed so much for. *I started off as a NQM at a large teaching hospital in a northern city, I hadn't trained there, knew nobody and had had a year off to have a baby. Despite this* ***on the first shift I was shown to a room to care for a high-risk woman in labour- literally nobody supported me or hardly spoke to me, I hadn't even been shown around!*** *I'd never read any of the Trust policies or had any Trust training by that time. I started my career terrified, unsupported and vulnerable. Even during emergencies,* ***I felt badly supported and blamed.***

A clear culture of bullying dominated labour ward, junior midwives were laughed at for pulling emergency buzzers or criticised for asking for help or even for expecting a second midwife at a birth - this had dangerous consequences. ***Later in my career I was a community midwife including in a CoC team. The on calls were crippling, expected to work all day and during the night with no limits, treated like a lesser human when called to labour ward with no support, no break*** *and told I couldn't leave if I stated that I was dangerously tired after working all day too, and then expected to drive safely home.* ***The lone working caused me anxiety going out alone day or night sometimes to areas or properties that were known to be high risk for lone workers and nobody checking on our well-being. Our on calls were nearly always into our day off so even our precious days off were often ruined - how is this ok to be on call into your days off when you deserve that break so much?***

One night I'd worked all day and then called into the unit straight away before going home, then went home for an hour before being called to a home birth, then at 06.30 (on my day off) they called to ask me back to the unit as I left the home birth - I refused and I was vilified for it- it's seen as some kind of dangerous badge of honour to work all day and night but god help the midwives that try and be safe and say when they're tired *- there needs to be legal limits and boundaries regarding on calls including not into your day off.*

CoC worries me tremendously as it does so many others- it's causing midwives to retire early and others to consider to leave but nobody's listening! Not all midwives want to work in all areas and that should be ok, midwives are being drawn into community from already dangerously under staffed maternity units - nobody wants a tired midwife who's worked countless hours looking after them - they want a rested, happy supported midwives experienced in the particular needs of that person.
My little dream is that on every shift there was at least one midwife completely impartial whose sole purpose was to support the needs and well-being of the staff, especially the junior ones, somebody any staff can call on to ask for advice to help with difficult situations as they happen, and regular opportunities for staff to speak with matrons about concerns without judgement. *Thank you for listening - this is just the tip of the iceberg of everything I could say."*

"I am currently looking for alternative jobs away from NHS midwifery due to stress and burnout, related to the staff shortages and workplace culture of my current Trust. *When I started as a student in 2015, we regularly had 20/21 midwives allocated to work across the floor (AN/PN wards, triage and delivery suite/MLU). However as is happening nationally, we are regularly running with such a low amount of staff that it is unsafe and unsustainable. Some shifts just 8 midwives across the floors. Midwives are constantly pulled to work on delivery suite. It is regularly now just 1 midwife allocated to care for every PN woman and baby on the ward. 1 Midwife allocated to every AN admission and PN readmission. 1 midwife in triage. The rest are spread to delivery suite and our MLU is forced to close, meaning our low-risk women are denied access to so many of their birthing preferences. It's heart-breaking. We spend shifts crossing our fingers that no spontaneous labourers come in as there is not a member of staff free to care for them. Inductions are told that we need to help deliver their baby early for whatever reason, but are then kept days waiting for IOL/ARM. We recently had a lady that had been in 10 days!* ***It is commonplace to see staff in tears and so many of us are looking for other jobs.*** *We cannot go on like this- being pulled from pillar to post, pressurised to swap shifts or do bank to cover shifts with crap staffing, regularly going 12.5 hours with no break. It is not safe for the people we care for and it is not safe for us.* ***It is not safe that we are encouraged to meet the needs of the service rather than the needs of those we care for.*** *It is not why I was drawn to midwifery. I go home days guilty and ashamed at the level of care given due to being stretched so thin. This cannot go on. Something must change."*

Blame Culture

Some midwives recounted how they were treated after an adverse incident, with little or no support, which led to them considering leaving midwifery.

"Earlier this year I was caring for a woman whose baby died shortly after birth due to bradycardia. It absolutely destroyed me as I had done everything I knew to do, there had been no indication of an issue until I struggled to find an FH and I was terrified of the repercussions. I was sent to eat something and organise somewhere to go when I left work before writing a statement. I was in the break room when the Head of Midwifery and 2 band 7s found me. I was distraught, crying, not making sense. ***The HOM looked me dead in the eye and told me someone had to be found to blame for what happened.*** *She'd never met me before. I was clearly devastated and blaming myself. I hadn't written my statement yet. I hadn't completed a full written retrospect. She didn't know the full story and*

she had already assumed I was to blame. I went on to develop severe anxiety and panic attacks over her words.

The band 7 in charge of the department took 5 days to phone me at home, when she told me, it wasn't my baby so why was I so upset. This band 7 is the same one who makes sure you know what happens in your room is your responsibility regardless of whether you ask for support. I was so glad I had a family bereavement the next day and a reason to be signed off sick for a few weeks other than a severe adverse event.

In all of this, the paediatric and obstetric staff were more supportive than the midwifery managers. It has completely changed my view of midwifery. ***There is blame in everything even when there is none.*** *It is always assumed and it is used to squash your spirit, keep you in line, make you live in constant fear. I dread how it would have been if I had made an honest mistake as do any of us really go to work to cause these traumas?* ***I'm now trying to leave the profession, as it has destroyed my mental health, relationships and life."***

"I trained in a mid-sized Trust that I joined in good faith after having positive birth experiences there. Initially, it was OK. ***There were a few hard-core senior midwives with a well-established clique and a Mean Girl attitude, but the HoM kept them mostly in check.*** *Then she left. Her replacement was vile, and she made it clear very quickly that she was not on our side.* ***The Mean Girls upgraded from 'you can't sit with us' to pushing others in front of a bus, and their culture was allowed to spread.*** *If you weren't in that clique, you couldn't professionally progress. You couldn't get breaks nor choose what area you wanted to work in. You couldn't finish on time or get the lighter workload.* ***The new HoM very much fed a blame culture, and guess who never got the blame?*** *Which left the rest of us constantly being micromanaged, berated and disciplined for misdemeanours that were excused and ignored in the clique.* ***Thankfully for me, I found a job in another Trust,*** *who have been infinitely more inclusive and supportive, and I've developed more as a midwife there than at my old hospital by far. However... the pressures on the service have proved to be fertiliser for incivility. I don't want to say bullying, certainly not at least 95% of the time, but there is now an undercurrent of bitching that wasn't there before. I'm now on a CoC team which I joined full of passion and excitement. It was working really well, and our stats supported that. Poor staffing levels have led to us increasing our caseloads, supporting other teams and most of all, frequently being used in escalation. When we first started, I would maybe be called in once in every 4 or 5 of my on-calls. Now it is the complete opposite, I get to stay home maybe 1 in 4 or 5. This means*

working a full day, sometimes the only day in the week that I have to see my own antenatal patients, often the only midwife in my team available for postnatal visits, then being called back in within 3 hours of getting home, or sometimes less. Then staying for up to 12 hours, which is actually the norm now. Despite this, preference seems to still be given to core staff for breaks, lighter workloads and finishing early (or even on time!). Everyone is on edge and our sickness rates are simply unreal, even allowing for COVID. I know core staff are struggling too, but it seems they forget that we worked a full day before we come in.

It makes everyone exhausted and narky, which naturally makes for an unpleasant and crucially *unsafe* working environment. *Which increases sickness, which makes it even harder for those working, which makes everyone narky... We're stuck in a cycle, and we haven't been given any hope for a way back. New preceptors are starting, but not as quickly as staff are leaving. I'm so scared for the new starters, how on earth will they cope when even those of us with experience can barely cope?* ***We are in crisis, and for the first time ever, I'm giving serious consideration to leaving the profession.*** *I never considered it when my old employers ground down my confidence and my trust. I never considered it when my personal circumstances made clinical work damn near impossible. But I'm considering it now. The only thing stopping me is knowing that my patients and my colleagues will suffer for it."*

D. Leave Midwifery and Move to Another Role in or Outside of Healthcare

Negativity and Lack of Positive Feedback

A lack of positive feedback and negativity contributed to these midwives leaving midwifery.

"It was then that I started looking for alternative roles. By the ***time I left maternity I was so ground down, felt like the worst midwife in the world."***

"I left midwifery last year after 16 years. *It was a mixture of feeling my skills were unrecognised, being bullied for the first time in my life, and realising that absolutely nothing would be done about it, and* ***the way we were treated during Covid, being told we were not allowed to wear PPE was a particular low point."***

"Have just left midwifery after struggling with run ins with a particular band 7."

Grieve for no longer being a midwife

Some of the midwives left, not because they wanted to but because they felt they had no option. These midwives described how they loved being a midwife and miss being one. One of the midwives describes the sense of loss as grief!.

"I knew I wanted to be a midwife from 13-years-old. Picked my GCSE and A-Level options based on that, resat a year because I was so determined I would manage it. Qualified at 22, managed just under 3 years before bowing out. I love my job now ***but I definitely grieve for the vocation that I dreamed of."***

"Slowly building myself up to applying for a bank contract to do the odd maternity shift again, but ***on my terms this time. I'm three years out of leaving my favourite role as a high risk midwife.*** *It was my dream, from age 11, to be one and I qualified aged 34."*

"I trained in a lovely unit but by the time I qualified things were going downhill and morale was low amongst the staff and our HoM who was fantastic, retired. I went to a new Trust with the majority of my cohort and loved it as a rotational midwife during my preceptorship. ***There was a handful of bullies but nothing I couldn't handle.*** *The unit was busy, big city, young population and births were booming.* ***The unit was like a factory, all I wanted to do was give the best care possible and treat women and their families with the respect they deserve and with that you need time.*** *I was often penalised for taking too long, for giving them a bed bath, for helping initiate breastfeeding before transfer to the ward for caring.*

Whilst on the PN ward the acting matron pulled me up on on-calls, we had to do one every 3 months and I had done my quota and questioned why I was put down for an extra one without my knowledge. *We self-rostered for these. That matron spent a good hour checking through what I had done over the past year, meanwhile I'm the midwife in charge of a busy PN ward with no staff. She undermined me in front of my colleagues and patients. I was so upset and this put me in a tizz for the whole long day shift but I did not let this effect my leadership or care.* ***She pulled me to her office as well to confront me as to why I wouldn't do it and was not able to comprehend I had done my quota and some midwives had not. I normally wouldn't kick up a fuss but it was a special occasion and I had made plans. Basically, she told me I had no choice I had to do it.***

The bullying continued the whole time I was rotating on that particular ward. My end goal was to be a community midwife, I absolutely loved it as a student. So, an opportunity came along and I took it. *Meanwhile the matron in community* *moved into a specialist role and this particular matron that did not like me swiftly moved in and made my life hell. Luckily my team lead was amazing and I didn't really have to go to the matron for much but there was always an atmosphere when we had protected time, social gatherings etc. I was quite often the on call with the home birth midwife. That horrible gut feeling never went, there was a lot of passive aggression but I ducked and dived as I found out I was expecting.*

After maternity leave, I knew I did not want to return to midwifery if working conditions didn't change. I wanted to be able to give the care that I wanted to give without being penalised! I'm now a health visitor and love it, it has its own stresses with staffing and caseloads but my team are brilliant. I would love to be a midwife again, I lived and breathed midwifery and worked so hard to get my degree, even with some bullies as students who excluded or ignored me. *If things don't change, I will never go back. Hats off to all the midwives continuing to give care and all the student midwives hanging in there."*

E. Left Midwifery

These midwives' accounts recall the bullying they were exposed to prior to leaving midwifery.

Bullied into Unnecessary Intervention

This midwife recounted feeling pressured into carrying out an intervention on a woman that wasn't necessary and left midwifery as a result, with no indication of the type of job she/he is working in.

"When I first left midwifery, my anxiety was sky high and I was afraid to post anything on this group in case said person was a member and I know colleagues are on here but now I'm getting better, I think sod it. Why should people get away with bullying? ***I'm so mad with myself that I let go some vicious comments made whilst at work, and allowed myself to perform an examination on a woman that was not necessary and didn't follow the Trust or NICE guidelines purely because I was being bullied into it by a coordinator, healthcare assistant and agency member of staff.*** *I don't think I will ever go back to midwifery which is a shame but I'm happy to fight for us as midwives for change."*

Working Conditions, Impacting Negatively on Standard of Care

The demands of the job were compounded by only being able to provide 'good enough' care as standard with midwives feeling that care was unsafe. A midwife with experience in other working environments was surprised that the bullying was not addressed.

"I loved my job *(as in the actual job itself) but there is* ***no way I could have faced sticking around with the way that everything else was going as it was overwhelmingly negative as well as emotionally, mentally & physically draining.*** *I think if I felt like I could do the job I love properly and give women good care then I probably wouldn't have left so soon, but it felt like that wasn't even an option any more.* ***Care was usually 'good enough' but that's not the midwife that I wanted to be."***

"There was bullying behaviour but in the main my mentors in community were fabulous and I knew I wanted to work there and work in a hands-on low tech environment. ***I never felt safe or that we worked at a safe capacity in hospital on the postnatal wards or on labour ward.*** *The first five years after training were the toughest and if it had not been that I had been doing a lot of community shifts and slotted in there immediately after my degree I do not think I would have remained in midwifery.* ***I could not believe the extent of the bullying culture that survived in the hospital particularly as I had already worked in private companies where staff would have been dismissed or reprimanded for the way they treated junior colleagues.*** *Wards could be a harsh tough place to work very much depending on who was in charge.* ***However, I loved my community job and even though like my colleagues, I regularly worked many hours overtime I had found my niche. Gradually the on call and pressure of caseloads took their toll and I decided to become part of the xx Programme believing that this could be a way for me to help improve the service.*** *We started work to caseloads of 30 to 32 which was brilliant and very satisfying however very quickly it became 35 36 and impossible to achieve a safe provision of care without working an impossible number of hours overtime. My sleep pattern became disrupted because of the high number of call outs and on calls and I eventually resigned from midwifery within the NHS. It has taken me most of a year and a half to return to a normal sleep pattern.* ***I am now working outside the NHS for a midwifery application with a great team and no levels of stress.*** *I think that midwifery within the NHS will break down eventually because it seems to becoming more and more short staffed. Plus,* ***I do not think the service will improve until the public are made truly aware of the stress that***

midwives undergo and the high burn out rates. *If there was one thing, I could see that would improve things is that community midwives and hospital midwives need to unite and appreciate that an across-the-board solution to lack of staffing needs to be found and an honest overhaul of public expectations and staff expectations discussed."*

"Where I trained there was low level 'cliquey' behaviour where if you were 'in' you would get first dibs on the shifts and who you worked with etc. Basically, however, it was mostly okay as a student and then as a NQM. I kept to myself and I was the one they would call on for the pool births (as others got backache...) and then I would support the VBACs with slightly 'off book' birth plans. I wasn't always 'in' but I wasn't 'out' either and I made it work and was basically respected as a good midwife and I know I had positive feedback from colleagues and students on many occasions.

I then moved Trusts and went straight to community and the attitude was not great. ***There was a lot (although not from all) of power play - both within the teams as well as towards women. It went all the way to management and I was asked, wrongly, to not work for a week after an incident (was all cleared after a few days and asked to come back...).*** *Nothing was dealt with properly and the incident was all down to the power culture and completely avoidable - no apology. I've left now and moved to a related area of care but did not feel safe - there was no teamwork if you were not one of the midwives that had trained and been there for years or were willing to sit and join in the disparaging remarks about the caseload.* ***The worst midwives were the ones who were then promoted. I can't imagine how it will change. On the surface they are all best buds and the best team but it's not real, there is no real woman-centred practice and it's all about ego and having the easiest life within the context of super short-staffing as they are in survival mode.*** *I can't understand the unkindness but I can see how the negativity perpetuates - the unit thinks community are 'soft' when that is very much not true, there are knee-jerk reactions to one-off events without thinking ahead or contextualising and perhaps doing more harm. It will only change when leaders and managers are empowered to show true empathy towards women and midwives. There needs to be enough staff at all levels and a culture of support and not fear."*

"I have recently left the profession as a band 7 Midwife. *Apart from the job changing beyond what profession I entered 13 years ago; I have never seen midwives so low in morale and no resilience left to fight because they are beyond exhausted.*

Aside from a very toxic culture which seems to be more and more widespread

across Trusts, the demands of the job, not just the expectations from DoH etc. but women themselves seem to be escalating beyond control, particularly fuelled by expectations of CoC. *I have never seen such poor mental health in a group of midwives. Personally, I didn't feel that I could lead a team when I had no faith in what those at the top are expecting of us.*

Sadly, there are a number of bullies within this profession which breaks my heart given that we are supposed to be part of a caring profession advocating for women.

I didn't see a way out other than leaving because I felt so broken that something had to give. *There is a huge crisis hitting Maternity services that needs immediate attention to ensure the safety of families."*

Targeted with Unfounded Allegations

Experiencing a range of bullying behaviours which then escalated into unfounded allegations about decision-making and care provided.

"My hellish experience of 3 years *will be difficult to condense into a short story but I'll try....*

I qualified as a midwife in xxxx and practised very happily for 15 years. I was very fortunate to work under amazing and inspirational leaders who cultivated and encouraged a passion for female empowerment, autonomy and midwife led care. I was always a midwife who enjoyed rotation as I enjoyed supporting women through their pregnancy journey into motherhood, and so was experienced in all settings. Their passion became my passion and I found myself wanting not just to advocate for women during pregnancy and birth but also for my colleagues who at times needed support in the workplace. I became a very active union steward, a role I enjoyed immensely discovering new talents I never knew I had. In the Trust I worked in at the time, I was very much nurtured, encouraged and supported to develop as was any midwife who showed a passion and initiative for improving the experience and care of women.

Although I never had any aspirations to progress in my career, senior management began to have quietly encouraging conversations asking that I give it some thought. Opportunities to progress in the Trust in which I worked at the time were limited and so in 2015 I ended up successfully applying for a management opportunity in a midwife led unit in a neighbouring Trust. Within 2 years my midwifery career was effectively over. *Naively I believed that all midwifery leaders were like those I had only ever known, how wrong I was. The undermining started off quite subtle*ty, primarily coming from another midwife manager, also newly *promoted. I had no idea it was happening at all until a woman I admitted to the unit in advanced labour birthed her baby without incident or difficulty, but baby's weight was below the 10th centile. As was the expectation, I completed a datix and informed the lead midwife only to find myself called to her office 2 days later and questioned about my decision making, care and qualifications for the job,* ***I had been in at this stage for 9 months. I was utterly gobsmacked and frankly left dazed and confused by what was happening.***

I suddenly found myself having to answer to other allegations and accusations and required to undertake an action plan. At the time, I had no difficulty at all doing this as I was always on a quest to improve and believed that all learning and self-reflection was a good thing. Although agreed by everyone, after 4 weeks merrily working towards the objectives agreed with and signed off by the senior managers, suddenly I was questioned again about the order in which I was following it and now being accused of avoiding addressing what they perceived as shortfalls in my midwifery experience. Next thing I was removed from post and sent to the main hospital of the Trust to be assessed.

The experience was horrendous and all but destroyed my confidence. *There were days when I was watched silently by 3 senior midwives as I provided care. Feedback was never positive with fault always found. I did not meet their expectations in the least and so was prevented from returning to my role. Once again, I was moved to another area to be scrutinised, still with no idea what I was doing wrong. 2 weeks later I received a visit from the lead midwife asking me how I was getting on to which I replied ok as I had been given no indication to think otherwise, only to be informed, I was being suspended from practice pending a supervisory investigation due to further complaints from midwives. This was later used as "evidence" of my lack of insight. No complaints from mothers were received I hasten to add, nor were there any incidents, datix reports, harm or detriment caused from any of the care I had provided. I was hit with 16 allegations, not all of which were practice related, and had a 17th thrown in at the end of a second supervisory interview.*

Having come from a background where I had gained lots of experience with assisting colleagues with statements for investigations of all level, I had a pretty good idea what to expect by way of process and procedure. ***Not a single procedure was followed the way it should have been. From the beginning, despite being a supervisory investigation, it was clear my 15 years' experience and suitability to meet the criteria for the job as it was originally advertised was being questioned.*** *I was effectively being accused of lying to get the job. Clinical records on the care I was being accused of not providing or inappropriately providing were not secured against which to question me, witness statements were not produced from* *my accusers and ultimately, when I was able to get my hands on records, which in all of the clinical cases disproved the allegation being made, I was told I was guilty based on the verbal accounts of recollections made by midwives, in some cases months after the event had occurred.* ***In each case as I was able to challenge the allegation, the allegation then would be changed to something else and in one particular case, when the evidence of the care medical colleagues alleged I had not provided was clearly documented in the woman's notes, I was told a handwriting expert would be required to verify it as two midwives, (not medical colleagues after all) verbally alleged I hadn't completed the assessment 6 months after the event.*** *The investigation including the production of a report took 9 months and despite being able to disprove most and in some where there was no evidence at all to support what was being alleged or that I was even present, I was found guilty of all allegations and told I would require a supervisory programme. I was on the verge of appealing the outcome, when I was told by the LSAMO that another HoM would gladly support me to undertake the programme in her Trust. This was 2017 and midwifery supervision was coming to an end soon.* ***By this stage I was utterly despondent, but still with a love for midwifery knew I had to find a way to regain my confidence and so reluctantly agreed to this as I knew I would be given a fair crack of the whip elsewhere. I did successfully appeal the process however.***

I was treated fairly as expected and 2 weeks into a 12-week programme was being asked by my programme facilitator why I was there. Reputed to be one of the hardest (but fairest) mentors to students and staff, she could find no fault with my practice. I exceeded the requirements of the programme but my employing Trust would not accept the outcome and would not allow me to return to my job. The union rep tried to question this decision but was ultimately stonewalled and for the first time I realised that the union I had belonged to for 18 years were without teeth and completely ineffectual. I was told I had to go back to the main unit which I refused on the basis I had been so traumatised by the previous experience I could not possibly practise and feel psychologically safe. So, I was sent to another unit within the Trust with no idea what to do or what was to happen. By this stage 15 months had passed since my removal from my original post, but despite this period of absence, ***I was told that due to staff raising fresh concerns about my practice, leadership and management style (to this day I don't know what those were) I was told the midwives had requested mediation which I had to participate in before I could return****. Again, I agreed with no difficulty, believing that colleagues should be prepared to do anything to improve relationships if that is causing issues for women in our care. We all believe ourselves to be good and decent human beings, but how we perceive ourselves in our own head and how others see us may not match.*

Although I never had a professional disagreement or difficulty with professional colleagues previously, I saw no harm in trying to understand the root of the issues this particular team had with me. Eventually after 2 months of waiting, and with my distress levels rising, I was invited to a mediation meeting. I was the only one there. I was told the mediator wanted to speak to me first. Puzzled as it was not what I was led to believe would happen I answered questions and engaged. The next meeting, a month later, was the same. No more meetings were planned and then I was told the midwives who supposedly had requested this process had withdrawn, essentially refusing to meet me face to face. *Again, details of the concerns being raised to justify being kept from returning to my post constantly changed.*

Each time I cleared the bar being set; the bar was raised. I was left in limbo in this unit not knowing what to do, what my role was or what next to expect when the answer came again and suddenly. ***I got a call from my union rep telling me further fault with my practice was found and I was to go off sick. I was told the union would be attempting to negotiate me out of my position and that if I did not consider a compromise agreement (a legally binding confidentiality agreement as I understand it to be) they would withdraw support.*** *I felt like I had been hit by a bus. It turned out what I was being accused of were minor documentation errors - not ticking a box, writing the wrong postpartum day in a diary although correct in the notes.* ***Although the same errors and sometimes more significant admin errors were made by colleagues, I was the only one ultimately put through a disciplinary process.*** *Not wishing any midwife colleague to experience this, or indeed be subjected to a formal investigation process but also trying to understand what was happening, I asked why I was being held to a different standard to my peers. I was then accused of trying to deflect blame and being incapable of taking responsibility.* ***2 weeks later I was told by a union rep, a person who I had held in high regard and respected all of my professional life, that my midwifery career was over.*** *This despite no NMC referral, no dismissal, not even a process started. It was simply the whiff of a possible blemish that would leave me unable to ever be trusted by a midwife colleague ever again and therefore best if I just retrained as something else at age xx. I was damaged goods now and no matter what happened, the midwifery world was too small to escape the doubt that would now always follow me she said.*

I fell apart, spiralled into depression, had thoughts of suicide and was eventually diagnosed with PTSD. I was full of self-doubt, questioned my sanity, personality and professionalism. Who was I? I did not recognise the person they were describing. *Was I really this awful person and so blinded by arrogance and conceit I couldn't see what an awful midwife I was? My relationships with friends* *and family were affected, I became a recluse and avoided the very town in which the maternity unit was located, terrified that I would come face to face with anyone part of it all. My waking mind was consumed by the torment, anguish, confusion and shame of what was happening and when sleep eventually came I was plagued by nightmares reliving the labour ward rooms over and over where I was being silently scrutinised by multiple managers.*

I was off sick for 5 months with the continual threat of formal suspension as I had refused to accept a confidentiality agreement which would have ended my career. *At one point after a lot of support from family and from previous trusted colleagues who knew me previously, I raised the possibility of a formal grievance as the concerns of my treatment which I had raised informally (2 folders worth of evidence) were ignored. My union rep had been supporting me with this and agreed to support it being made formal. However, after writing 2 drafts and sending it for review and submission, having not received any response I submitted it via the Trust portal which was what the process required. Suddenly I was called to a meeting with my union reps and told they were withdrawing support as I had contravened their contract with me acting independently of them. The document hadn't reached HR due to some glitch but, despite me offering to withdraw it so they could submit it, I was flatly refused and told no.*

When I eventually returned to work realising, I could no longer sit and wait for what I believed would be a formal suspension and an NMC referral, I found that this in fact did not happen and I was temporarily redeployed to wait the outcome of a Trust investigation into me and the outcome of my grievance. This took another year to complete, the outcome of which was my removal from post and a down-banding. I was however told I could practise as a midwife within the Trust maternity service (the irony has not escaped me), the rationale for which my union did not question given the "concerns" about my practice and decision making. I did not return to practice and instead remained in the redeployed role where I had felt supported as part of a reasonable adjustment for PTSD. I simply couldn't go back – the trauma was much too great.

During the long and protracted period of waiting for progress on the process, in a state of distress I had spoken many times of my willingness to self-refer to the NMC as I was beginning to believe that I must be a danger to women and wanted desperately to understand and take whatever action was needed to remedy my shortcomings rather than be a risk to any woman. This was always dismissed by my union. ***Much later during a conversation with my new senior manager also responsible for professional regulation in the Trust, I learned that the assistant director to whom I had submitted the grievance had on 3 occasions approached her to review my case for referral to the NMC. She had refused each***

time as the lead midwife and maternity staff had no evidence to support any of the allegations, it was, she said, all based on rumour, gossip and speculation. Learning this did not make me feel better. I felt incredibly let down by my union who did little to challenge anything but seemed more concerned with protecting their reputation and relationship with managers.

Earlier this year I worked a few bank shifts as a midwife in a Trust I had previously worked in and where I had always found the staff and management to be very supportive. They were incredibly understanding of my anxiety and did support me as best they could after a 3-year absence, but ultimately I'd lost faith. The flashbacks, feelings of distress and panic every time I walked into a labour room were just too overwhelming.

I have since moved on, completed a masters, and am retraining for another role within the health service. Writing my dissertation on "Why do midwives leave the profession/workforce prematurely" and the attempt to work the occasional midwifery bank shift led to the ***triggering of my PTSD and anxiety that I thought I had resolved so I'm back in treatment as ultimately I do not want the trauma to rule my life and future.***

I mostly have good days now. I get the occasional flashback and panic attack, but there's not a day goes by when I don't mourn the loss of a life that I loved. *It was a life I started in my 20s and I will always remember those amazing midwives from my first 15 years who laughed with me in my youthful exuberance, celebrated with me when I got married, shared their wisdom with me when I had children, and cried with me when I lost loved ones.*

Sadly, it is a life I can never return to but hope that my story will also contribute to culture change for the sake of the midwifery profession and women."

"I was bullied by a new jealous, sociopathic manager in 2015, and very many happy years in my Profession. *I was an enthusiastic, highly skilled, and popular midwife at a xx hospital, and she hated this.* ***I wasn't the only midwife targeted by her, but she went to town on me.*** *She made my life absolute hell, and I had time off sick. This was then used to organise a Disciplinary Sickness Absence Meeting, where I was very badly advised by the RCM (the woman was friends with my bully), to hand in my notice, which I did. I then did bank at another hospital, but within a few months, she then got the top job of Consultant Midwife there, and got me out super-fast. She eliminated me from NHS Professionals. It was as if I had never existed! I was Midwife to my daughter at the first hospital. Just my daughter, her husband and me, throughout the whole birth experience. She laboured in water, and came out for birth, as it seemed a large baby (9 and a half pounds!) Slight* *shoulder dystocia, completely dealt with by her husband getting her in McRoberts. This inspired my daughter to study midwifery, and she graduated with a First, and started work at my first hospital a year ago. She left after eight months, never to return. She now works in a delicatessen. Absolutely no support for newly qualified midwives, she never even had an exit interview!* ***What a total mess the Midwifery Profession now is. I really feel there is utterly no hope anymore."***

Bullied by Known Bully

This midwife felt that she had no option but to leave, having been bullied by a known bully.

"I left midwifery a year ago after 12 years of working at the same Trust. I experienced bullying from a more experienced midwife who was also known to bully other midwives and is now a matron at another Trust (despite complaints being lodged against her). *I had a band 7 trying to bully me as a newly qualified on delivery suite and I didn't feel supported. One of the midwives actually apologised to me after completing my preceptorship paperwork with me, she said 'you've been left to sink or swim, thank god that you swam'. The upshot being that after a year, I had anxiety and panic attacks. I carried on though, I had a family to feed and bills to pay and once settled into a community team after my preceptorship, I finally felt like my confidence and happiness was returning.*

Fast forward 10 years, ***a few more incidents of bullying, my love of the job had gone, morale was at an all-time low, CoC discussions were going on, midwives were saying 'it won't work' but we basically got told 'tough, that's how it is'. I looked for a different job and left before the 'shit hit the fan' so to speak.*** *I was very lucky to find a job where I can still use my skills and I work in a team where I'm trusted, my opinions are valued and I feel respected. ... what an absolute breath of fresh air that was to me. I still talk to friends who work there and they say midwives are leaving by the droves, no one is happy, staff are completely demoralised and beaten down.* ***It's so sad, I'd have happily have finished my career there as a midwife if I'd have been valued more."***

Bullied as a Midwife and Received Poor Care as Woman

This midwife experienced poor care during labour and birth, suffered from Post-Natal depression as a result and then returned to the same Trust to work as a midwife, only to be bullied and experience sustained poor working conditions.

"I gained employment with the Trust that contributed to my birth trauma. Left naked, covered in blood and faeces after a forceps birth and haemorrhage I was abandoned with no food, forced to crawl to the toilet to empty a leaking bladder, as blood poured from me. I did this as an experienced midwife hearing the emergency buzzers going on the delivery suite I was required to stay on for close observation. Observation that did not occur because the midwives were over stretched and overwhelmed by a system failing the staff and clients.

I went on to work at the Trust for 10 years despite severe postnatal depression, anxiety and sleep deprivation. Forced to work enforced overtime to be on call for the unit that just being near gave me panic attacks as I was triggered by my own birth trauma.

For 10 years I battled with bullying, coercion, severe understaffing and my requests for additional training blocked. *I worked over my hours and never had a lunch break just so that I could fulfil my duties knowing I was never giving what my clients deserved and that I was complicit in the same sort of birth trauma that I had experienced myself.*

Following a miscarriage, I was interviewed by Occupational Health for my absence and told to "prepare for the worst" i.e. being fired, and then forced to wait 8 weeks for a meeting with the Matron. Those 8 weeks caused immense stress and uncertainty. When meeting with the Matron, I was questioned about my need for leave and offered no sympathy when I explained I bled for 2 weeks waiting to pass my dead baby. I was then "invited" to resign but (through tears) told her if she wanted rid of me, she would need to fire me and prepare for the legal action I would take.

I experienced severe neglect and eventually became suicidal. My resilience was constantly questioned and the blame shifted. Even after returning to work, when they knew I had been suicidal my phased return was denied.

I have now left the Trust to fulfil a non-clinical role to my great relief. However, I'm angry for the 10 years I was forced to live in fear, for the cost on my family, my mental health and the chronic, stress related physical illness I am now left with for the rest of my life as a result. I am grateful to those colleagues who supported me. I wish for a better environment for them and for the families under their care. ***The system broke me as a birthing person & a midwife. I'm forever changed.*** *I don't want anyone else having to survive what I did. In love, admiration and solidarity to all those still practising."*

Negative Impact on Health and Well-Being

A couple of midwives made it clear that they left due to the negative impact of bullying on their health and well-being.

"For 13 years I have been qualified as a midwife and since leaving the profession I have commenced counselling for PTSD from my experience. ***I'm so glad I left, during the whole of my career I've witnessed bullying and unprofessional behaviour not always directly to myself but to others but not felt able to stand up for them.*** *This is one of my many regrets. I've began to realise that maybe the women were bullied as well, were they made to feel guilty for their choices because it didn't suit that midwife or did they experience this unprofessional behaviour between staff or between staff and students? How is that ok?*

The Trust I worked for was the typical "face fit" culture. *If your face didn't fit then your opinion was ignored, you were laughed at if you wanted to make change, if you applied for a job, you wouldn't get it not because of your experience or your interview technique but because you weren't the person the management wanted. If you asked for feedback, you wouldn't get any. Frequently staff would hear the interview panel bragging that they could pick who they wanted for jobs and that the other people shouldn't even bother attending. You couldn't go to anyone because the management was part of the problem, or were deluded by the senior bullies who knew exactly to get around them. Most would do very little work and would sit on their phones calling their families or on FB. They would openly moan if you pressed the emergency bell, and if things resolved, accuse you of being a terrible midwife who was no good. Would then tell everyone at the desk and if they didn't agree they would be branded a s**t midwife too.*

Each part of the department hated each other, no one worked as a team. You could be a labour ward midwife one day and then be rotated to community and, if you phoned to transfer someone in to the labour ward, staff would no longer believe you saying "well are you sure" "you are a community midwife now". As if this makes you less competent! Students are frequently found crying as are newly qualified staff. Before I left more and more staff were leaving, it became unbearable to work there. Staff including myself were crying daily. New staff were employed to attempt to fill the many posts available and they were bullied from the moment they started rather than welcomed. Branded as useless before they've even done anything. Managers allowed it to happen, they allowed those bullies to have what they wanted regarding off duty, rotation and promotion and everyone else was told they would have to be redeployed, they signed a rotational contract or maybe they shouldn't be a midwife.

Continuity teams commenced with staff at an all-time low, not surprisingly it failed. Those in the teams tried their best, it was painful to watch. They were broken. Not because continuity won't work but because the management and the senior staff bullies didn't support it, didn't staff it and left the workforce to burn out and then blame them for the lack of achievement.

I have a new job and my employer cares about me as a person, that on its own is hard to come to terms with. *I realise now I will never go back. Being a midwife has taught me many things but the biggest thing is life isn't always predictable and we should embrace the things that make us happy. Sometimes it means we have to make hard choices like leaving our career. My last shift was hard, very few people cared. I drove away feeling hurt and betrayed but then I realised when my time comes to leave this Earth, I will see my life out before me and I will be proud and content with the choices I made. I know I never bullied anyone and if I had a bad day I always apologised if I snapped. I supported those who asked for my help. My only regret is not standing up to the bullies. Maybe just writing this will be some form of help in changing the future."*

"Until March this year I was an NHS Nurse and Midwife. *I worked and loved my role for 20 years but after a horrific year of* ***watching myself and my colleagues suffering the most appalling bullying I left.*** *I am currently still receiving support for the trauma* ***but I am now working for an employee that values me and pays me well.*** *What most concerned me about this incident, is that despite numerous reports of bullying and harassment and unsafe staffing to even the chief executive, nothing was done. I would also add that despite contacting head of HR and CEO, I never even received a response. I never received even a leaving card or acknowledgement of my many years of service. Neither did my colleagues. Such a terrible waste of valuable experienced staff that are not easily replaceable.*

I didn't realise how it had affected my mental health until I was in a terrible state. Now gone it has made me reflect how much better I feel and how wrong it was. *It's like it's gone backwards! When I was a student nurse, I would have been horrified had I witnessed the inhumane behaviour not just to staff but to patients also."*

This is an account from an MSW who eventually left, because of the impact on her health, including suicide attempts, and is retraining in another role in healthcare.

"In 2018 I was an MSW working in the community in my normal day 5 and breast-feeding clinic. I was sadly presented with a day 5 baby who had a dusky episode. The baby needed resuscitation, I was on my own with a mobile phone

and 2 hysterical parents. It resulted in me giving 1 breath for the baby to respond and then I called 999. *The Paramedics arrived after 10 minutes so I had a dusky baby and 2 screaming parents begging me to help. The baby was blue lighted into hospital. On that day I was asked to write a statement. For weeks after I was put on a pedestal by my management team and HoM until they received a complaint from the parents. They accused me of lying and that I did not resuscitate their baby. My management team responded to the parents supporting me. And told me not to worry. It ruined my Christmas. In February, 3 months after the episode I received a text message by my team leader who is also a very good friend. She asked me to come into the unit for an informal meeting with the deputy HoM and the HoM. I contacted my union rep who contacted HR as I felt something wasn't right. HR reassured them that there were no meetings they were aware of and to attend the meeting with support.*

When I got into the unit, I was refused support from the deputy HoM and taken to the HoM's office. I have been in the NHS for 25 years and I have never been in any situation like this. Once in the HoM's office I was refused representation again when I asked and I was suspended on the spot. *I must add HR were not present and were not made aware of the meeting. I was allocated one of the HoM's management team to be investigating officer. I was asked to hand over my mobile my lap top my badge and my carpark pass and then I was walked off the premises as I was supposedly not safe to be working with children.* ***I was sent a letter within 4 days stating not to communicate or contact anyone in the NHS and I could not leave the area without the HoM's approval. This meant I had no support or contact and I could not visit my ill family member or my family as I am 200 miles away from them. This was the first time I tried to end my life.***

Fast forwarding the HoM in her statement accused me of having fabrication of illness by proxy. Her episode of suspension was not included in my meeting as it was said to be a separate investigation to my grievance and I was dismissed from my post. ***My second attempt of suicide came shortly after. I had to let my son live with his dad and I had to go into a debt consolidation which I have for 6 years.***

With help from friends and family and policies I proved my innocence. *It came to light that the recording of the 999 call, and the ambulance report concluded that I was factual and transparent in my statement. All investigating officers and managers heard and read this report but it was kept from me. In xxxx, I won my job back.* ***When I returned I was made to feel I still did wrong as they would not allow me to go back to community and I was treated so differently to others by having to shadow and work on a ward I finally decided for my mental health to leave.***

I learned from the investigation my team leader/ friend was forced to send the message to me on that day and was threatened with her job if she prepared me for what was about to happen. They used her as they knew I trusted her. Today that baby is fit and well but I still struggle a little working with children and working alone. ***I left the hospital to get away from it.*** *I am currently 2 years into my debt recovery and my son is home with me. And finally I am at university training to be a xxx.* ***The CEO personally apologized to me and asked how she could reach out to other staff to stop the bullying culture she was aware of. There is still bullying but I hope my brave actions fighting against it, has given others a voice to stand up for themselves."***

F. Staying as Need to Work

These midwives' accounts recount how they have been exposed to a range of bullying behaviours, including preferential treatment for other midwives, cliquey behaviour and poor working conditions have made staying in midwifery difficult. Some of the bullies appear to be untouchable as they work for a workplace union. Bullying in academic workplaces is also highlighted. However, these midwives have stayed, some have changed jobs but need to stay in work and and for personal reasons cannot leave.

Persistent Bullying that is Not Addressed

This account is about the lack of action by the employing Trust even in one case when an incident of physical assault was reported to the Police. Also, accounts of the bully being promoted and the complaints not being addressed.

"During the first week of my second year student placement, I found a 28/40 (28 week pregnant) woman having decelerations down to 60bpm for around 60-90 seconds and completely unprovoked. The mum was being tested for pre-eclampsia but not yet diagnosed. The baby was born by GA an hour later and went home at 35 weeks. ***My mentor never praised me and in fact told me I'd never qualify as I wasn't "midwife material". This same midwife went on to become my manager who then questioned my ability to be a midwife due to being newly diagnosed as hypoglycaemic. Again, this was clearly rubbished this time by my consultant and occupational health.***

Then the real nightmare, she became matron. I was physically assaulted at work by a staff member and I went to my manager who did nothing, then her as matron who also did nothing so I involved a workplace union who said report it

to police as a common assault which I did. The Police then obviously got involved with my Trust and their lack of doing anything about it and they warned the colleague.

After this I had midwives who didn't even know my ward, to come over and be in charge of the ward, the MCAs told me they had been told to write down anything I had to leave or I'd have become more mentally unwell than I was feeling. ***For 15 years, I have been bullied by this one woman who has abused her power over me from day one and she's just gone further and further up the ladder."***

Bully Seems Untouchable

"My input is fairly simple:

What do you do when the bully has made herself almost untouchable? *A midwife for several years AND has a role within the Union. The repercussions for the person reporting this bullying (and their future in midwifery) feel immense, who would want to stand up against someone with a position within the Union and have the perpetrator bad mouth you to their peers?*

I know of others who have been significantly ***bullied by midwives who are xxx Union reps****. It seems becoming a rep, or higher within the Union, is a way for bullies to protect themselves by ingratiating themselves with the very union who should protect midwives from bullying.*

I would also like to add that most Union reps I've met are wonderful and caring midwives who are there to support us. I know they will be shocked and saddened by what I've written.

It just feels like my bully protected herself from any accusations by being a rep, or gaining a higher position within the union, and this is also true of other people who've confided in me about the bullying they've had and have felt unable to report it because of the bully's position.

Bullying in Academic Settings

Midwives attending University on a post graduate course felt bullied by the lecturing staff.

"There is a world crisis for midwives and in a country which prides itself in its level of health care, it's shocking that there isn't care for the young midwives. It's really shocking. I returned to do a post-grad 6 month module some years ago and ***I was so shocked at the bullying churned out to my colleagues by other colleagues who happened to have trained at the same time as most of us. They were the teachers/***

lecturer but without exception the class knew more but were treated as total fools... *No wonder the system is rotten. It's the same all over I have seen it in so many countries... How to change this or even deal with it is so exhausting.... We so need kindness in our world, kindness everywhere.*

Preferential Treatment and Not being Listened to

This midwife highlights the cliques and preferential treatment afforded to some midwives. Also levels of staffing meant that it was difficult to ensure that mothers and babies were given the care they needed with midwives being told that there was nothing could be done about the staffing levels.

"I nearly left midwifery while still training as I was dealing with racism at placement and general bullying from a lot of the midwives *(as many students were also suffering). This triggered my anxiety in an alarming way and every shift started and ended with dread and tears. I was penalised for supporting other students who were seen to be issues and I was warned several times that my association with these students was going to make my life difficult. My final year was the worst and definitely had me considering some awful things and I'm honestly surprised I made it through.*

When I qualified, I almost didn't feel joy but at least knew I'd have some relief. When I started my new role, I was apprehensive but had moved to a new area and was finally about to start the job I had worked so hard for. ***The culture of bullying, the cliques, the preferential treatment of midwives who were seen by many as lazy, and the bending of policies surrounding safe care time and time again has taken its toll and on my very worst shift I was left with one midwife and 2 MSWs for a full postnatal ward (20 women and babies) of complex medical and social cases. We escalated several times, begging for help and was told there was nothing that could be done.*** *We were transferred another woman even when we had said we couldn't safely take her and found that she had already been brought to the ward and settled in a bay. When I queried it with the shift coordinator, who had snuck her in, and made clear we were overwhelmed and couldn't provide care for her, she simply replied, "you'll be fine". The pressures of the shift took its toll and by the time I managed to get to this woman, she was sobbing in pain and her partner was shouting threats at me down the phone. He later came to the ward looking for me and only then were our pleas listened to and the coordinator finally came and transferred her back to labour ward, where she should have been the whole time. I was ridiculed for being scared of the partner.*

I thought this was my dream job but honestly, with the way things are

currently and have been for a while, I'm unsure as to how long I can stay with it like this. I'm worried for students and the quality of the education they're getting; I'm worried for all NQM because they aren't getting the support they deserve; *I'm worried for our experienced midwives because the burnout from trying to bridge the gap for support for everyone while getting their own work done is killing them and I'm worried for the families accessing the service. Something has to be done.* ***We're not paid enough; the work life balance is non-existent and our working conditions are dangerous."***

I've never known anything like it, the workload and hours are enough and we would pull together and get the job done, ***but the added complexity of such a toxic substandard leadership makes you feel like you are so insignificant and worthless, I feel like I've wasted 7 years of blood, sweat and tears because I've been completely stonewalled and denied opportunities. There's a definite elite group who are in the matron's pocket and the development and progression is exclusive to them.***

I worked at the Trust where I trained and as a student knew who the bullies were but never had any real issues. ***After 2 years I became pregnant and that's when I started to experience bullying from my team leader and matron.*** *My team leader would not sign my leave form and she would not give me my annual leave but kept trying to assign it when she wanted me to have it. I thought by speaking with the matron as my team leader advised me to would help but it got worse and I had to go to the union rep. That's when all hell broke loose and I ended up going on mat leave early due to the stress of my leader giving me horrendous tasks to do, no safety checks or anything.*

On my return I was lied to and told that my team no longer had space and therefore I had to go elsewhere and, when I made a fuss and said that I knew the team was actually short, they gave me another Team covering an area that was extremely far from my childcare which I'd arranged with the fact that I was still breastfeeding and I wanted to be in the same area in mind. *I told my matron this and she said "Well your child is 1 now so she should be eating food". I wish I was exaggerating but that's what she said. I was given a very busy clinic and was told* ***I could express my milk in the dusty stationary cupboard or the tiny kitchen, there wasn't even anywhere to store my milk.*** *I went on to have mastitis twice and when my child got chicken pox after I was back for only 3 weeks, I took 2 days off and, on my return, I was taken into a meeting with the new team leader and same matron and told that this cannot happen again and I should have arrangements in place for my child (I did hence why I was back after 2 days). I* ***went on to have postnatal depression of which I hid until after my 2nd child and I still suffer***

Working Conditions and Racism

These midwives recount their experience of poor working conditions, favouritism and experiences of racism

"Midwife with over 30 years' experience.

I've just got in from the shift from hell and I want to quit. *I was rostered to work on the MLU but got there and it was in darkness - there was a note.*

Hi, can you please go to ....and support for the late shift, many thanks x

So, I went. The postnatal ward. 24 beds. 4 bays of 4 and then 8 single rooms

One band 5 midwife had turned up for work this morning.

So, a band 6 from another ward went to 'support' her.

She went home at 3pm, I started at 3pm. So, no handover time. I had 3 bays - she had the rest - some were COVID positive - and quite poorly

66% of mine were sections - all less than 48 hours - most were primips, all wanted to BF - all were topping up

Some hadn't had pain relief since 0100 in the morning

Some hadn't been out of bed, washed etc

It was a shambles

And when I asked the delivery suite co-ordinator to let us have a MW for the drugs round - the MW was bringing another patient who had had a section up (and the baby wasn't going to survive), she said no - none of her staff had had breaks - this was at 1830.

When I told her my staff hadn't either she said we should have.

Then rang back 5 mins later - phone answered by MSW who was told the co-ordinator wanted to speak to the midwife- but not me! ***She then proceeded to shout at the band 5 midwife screaming why you haven't had your break.***

And then the band 5 started crying!

The husband of the woman in room x started shouting where was his wife's medication and his daughter's blood results; the man in one of the bays needed to know if the baby shaking was normal; and the woman in bed A2 was sobbing as her baby is on NNU and getting worse and no one listened when she asked for steroids before her elective section; the women in bed A2's nipple was chewed off by her baby because she was struggling on her own

And I lost the BP machine (found later in the xx - no idea why I left it there!)

Left the ward in tears at 2100hr after shift finished at 2000hrs

I've never felt so useless in my life. I've been doing this job for over 30 years. It was dire.

And the staff are all worn down. I called the bed manager down to complain. She said what can I do? There are no midwives.

They know there is a bullying culture on the delivery suite - and are trying to address it - but it's horrendous.

Ethnically I was in the minority. I had not experienced anything like it before in my general nurse training or working as a staff nurse. *Labour ward staff were the worst insisting in calling the students by their last name only and working us hard all through the shift and often long after. No breaks or comfort stops were allowed. As soon as one delivery was completed you were moved into the next room often just catching the baby without really knowing or learning anything. It was all about getting your 40 deliveries as quickly as possible to the staff, so you didn't require so much supervision. I was not the person then that I am today and didn't speak out at the time. I've worked in many Trusts since and again there are senior staff managing the shift who try their hardest to intimidate you and question your experience. We have all been given the primip on Synto to care for but some students and junior midwives are given these patients for every labour ward shift, day or night.*

There is a culture of "in my gang" that monopolises the staff. It often starts at the top with the managers/matrons and continues amongst senior midwives. *I have known senior staff request off duty of junior staff and students be changed so they don't have to work with them.* ***Staff are ostracised, demoralised often publicly humiliated in-front of others or women and their families.*** *Snide remarks are made and don't get me started on WhatsApp groups. Nothing has changed in 35 years.* ***I have remained in midwifery and continue to try and make a difference to the staff I work with caring for families.***

The HoM who bullied me and caused my heartache has just been promoted to a position at the xxx! Just goes to show the bullies get rewarded. *She ruined the careers of a few midwives in xxx and xxx. So if it's rotten at the top where do we go from here? Midwives approached her and told her we were on our knees, to which she replied we can always replace you. I hope with all my heart that change will happen but I'm not naive to the politics of what that would mean. Scotland is as bad as England."*

"I qualified in 2011 and have been actively practising ever since. I have worked community, postnatal/antenatal ward, and mostly delivery suite in my time. A couple of years ago I landed my dream job... a specialist role that I had been dreaming of for over 10 years. The kind that, even as a student you think 'one day I'll be in that role'. It was in a trust I'd never worked at before so I wasn't familiar with the characters there, you know the usual 'who to avoid, and who you can approach'. I was so excited to start this role but it became very clear right from the first day I set foot on delivery suite that I was going to have an issue with a

particular co-ordinator. ***There's history as to why she singled me out which I won't go into as it would make me identifiable.*** *From day one she's been openly rude to me, she publicly picks holes in everything I do or don't do and rallies up other staff against me, to align them to her point of view.* ***She sends openly rude, inappropriately critical emails - I'm at a point where I feel physically sick every time her name pops up in my inbox. The worst part of this is that the management know about it.*** *She CCs in the matrons when she sends me nasty emails on occasion - and though they will then verbally say to me that it's not ok for her to speak to me like that, they then don't have the confidence to challenge her on it. On one occasion she spoke to me so appallingly it was all I could do not to cry - this happened in front of a band 8, who told the deputy HoM about it. I happened to be alone in an office with the same deputy HoM later that day (leaving at 7pm after a clinic that should've finished at 5) and she didn't even ask me if I was ok, let alone ever do anything about it. And why does no one challenge her on this behaviour? Because 'that's just how she is'...'****oh her women love her, she gives them her all'...'she's just passionate about the subject.' No. She's a bully. She has me scared to walk in to delivery suite for fear of what I'm going to have to deal with, what I'm going to have to pretend doesn't hurt me,*** *how I'm going to have to justify myself to her today.* ***I've never been a wallflower; I've always stood up for myself and I consider myself resilient but this experience has ruined a dream that I have had ever since I started my training.*** *I can't understand why this behaviour is still considered acceptable so thank you for speaking out and starting this movement."*

"Life as a midwife of colour is not easy at all. *I have been reading the anonymous posts and at the same time I realise that the majority of midwives here are Caucasian, midwifery itself remains a largely Caucasian dominated profession. The stories being posted here are horrific and extremely painful to read. When I read some of them, I am literally reliving some of my past. As I am reading some of inhumane and torturous experiences some of have been forced to go, I can't avoid asking myself this one question, if this is what Caucasian midwives are going through, then what are the rest of us (midwives of colour) are going through?* ***Most of what midwives of colour have experienced will never be known because we are generally quite voiceless, seen as insignificant.*** *Personally, family and faith have kept me sane, if I had not been brought up in a country that has once experienced both apartheid and genocide* ***my experience in midwifery would have sure led me to committing suicide, because yes, I have been down a very dark path****. I keep telling myself I survived genocide and apartheid and so nothing really should upset me. But hey I am human, and to be honest the apartheid and genocide were* *probably less traumatising, because the mental turmoil I have personally gone through is unbearable! I have become morbidly obese from work related stress and this has led to infertility. I have developed panic attacks which I never had ever, I have zero confidence and other health issues.* ***I truly hate my job. I cry a lot in my sleep when these things come to my mind. I will one day have the courage to write about my gruesome and cruel experiences as a midwife.***

Feeling Suicidal

"In 2016, I was a full time Community midwife working in a team in a low-socioeconomic area, many asylum seekers, high Asian/Czech, non-English speaking. High rates of Domestic Abuse, housing issues, high mental health rates, social involvement. I was never afforded any extra time to attended Child in Need (Safeguarding) meetings, any extra time for interpreting. The amount we were spending on interpretation services was frowned upon. Antenatal appointments were 15 minutes long and 1 hour for booking often complex needs.

I initially enjoyed my work here and felt I supported the women well. *My name got round the community and women often asked for me by name to join my caseload. The team was quite disjointed and went through many different staff in the 3 years I was with this team. Staff often went off with mental health issues after only a short time with us.* ***Our workload was so high, we heavily depended on students to get round all the women we needed to see. I'm not proud of the pressures we put these students under.*** *We went through 4 line managers in the time I was there.*

It was in 2016 when ***after a short time the newly appointed admin assistant took a great dislike to me. She claimed she was very friendly with my manager.*** *She seemed to feel as I took time with my women that I wasn't working as hard as the rest of the team. Part of my coping would be to grab my lunch at a local ASDA and one day prior to my A/L I popped in to buy lunch and saw a t/shirt I would like to buy near the cash desk. This particular day, I had taken some visits from another team close to my home, so signed out of my base an hour early so to fit the 3 visits in on my way home. She took this opportunity (with proof) to insinuate I had left early but still claimed extra time on my time sheet. I was called in for a meeting with my manager about my time management and falsification of my time sheet.* ***My manager accused me of claiming time I wasn't working. She also accused me of falsifying the amount of visits I had.*** *I was absolutely beside myself and told her she could have my diaries and check notes for herself.*

I didn't hear anything else and shortly after she left as my manager and her best friend became my manager. From that moment on I felt hounded. I was rung several times during the day to see where I was and what I was doing. She would send me pointless emails requiring answer to see how often I accessed my emails. She would "delegate" menial tasks that in my view that were her role not mine. In the last 4 months I was there, a new band 6 midwife commenced. She was incredibly lazy and would often come on late often after early morning duties had been undertaken and say she had to leave early on several occasions a week for various reasons. Another colleague of mine brought this up with her on several occasions. Eventually this midwife made a complaint about the two of us, stating she felt bullied by us, when I felt I done everything to support her, whilst I was swimming with workload and harassment from my manager and lack of team members.

My work started to suffer and a complaint went in from one of my ladies, stating she felt I had no empathy for her, she rang me 30 minutes prior to her appointment every time with several excuses why she couldn't attend. *On the last appointment I offered her a later appointment and she started shouting at me over the phone telling me "you're supposed to be the one". The expectation of the women had become unrealistic of me. My managers expectations had become unrealistic. My colleagues were taking advantage of my work ethos. I was taking more and more on but I was being made to feel like I couldn't do enough. I was made to feel like I was a problem.* ***I was belittled in front of members of support team and I was belittled by the support team due to institutional bullying.*** *Students who worked with me often commented how busy I was and how much extra workload I took on.*

One day I had worked with a StMW who had worked as an MSW. She was in her 2nd year. We had had a pretty stressful day. I was in early, I had the majority of visits, many women were upset and needed extra input. I was late off without a dinner break. The student's eyes were widened as she couldn't believe just how much work we had undertaken that day. She finished by saying she felt she was going to gain so much experience and thanked me for an enjoyable day and for being so kind. The next morning, I walked into the office to find her crying. I took her to another room. She told me she had been harassed that morning by our MSW and ward clerk on what we had actually done yesterday. ***She stated their tone was awful and they insinuated I was lazy and hoped she wasn't learning to be lazy too. She was so upset as she knew this just wasn't true. She said the way they talked about me was so disrespectful. She knew awful lazy midwives and she knew I wasn't one of those.***

I was at my lowest point now. I shut down. I was paranoid. ***My self-worth had been battered out of me. I had no self-confidence and my sense of self was rock bottom. I wasn't good enough!*** *In my 2 hour appraisal I sat with my manager* *where she berated me, put me down, told me I had a wicked tongue in my head, told me I was a good midwife but there was just a nasty side to me. I asked to be transferred into the unit as I had had enough.* ***She told me, "don't think you can escape from me into the unit". I just sat there. I had no fight left.*** *She took great delight in telling me she had finally received a complaint from a woman and told me she was onto me. The next morning, I was so upset at the thought of another day at work, I was thinking of ways I wouldn't have to go. My thoughts were racing and fleeting and before I knew it, I was performing an emergency stop with a brick wall an inch away from my car. It took me a few moments to realise what had just happened.* ***I had purposely attempted to drive my car into a wall to avoid going into work that day.*** *I sobbed all the way into the office with the help of a friend over my hands free (she wanted to get me somewhere safe). I attended the office where my 1 supportive colleague was there. I rang my manager and told her what had just happened. Her reaction was stern "and what do you want me to do about that"! I was beside myself and broke down. My colleague came and I'm not really sure what happened after that. I do remember feeling numb, helpless numbness. I sobbed and wailed like a mother whom had lost a child. I was grieving. My partner had to come collect me from work that day. I was taken to the GP.* ***Where I admitted I had planned 3 different ways in which to kill myself because of my job.*** *I had stock piled Codeine from when I broke my coccyx and another strong pain relief and paracetamol. I had thought of giving myself an air embolism with equipment from my Homebirth bag and attempted to drive into a wall at high speed.*

So that was that. I was off work for 5 months, all the time harassed to come back by my manager. OH suggested I come back into the unit due to the amount of on calls and hours I was working and the harassment I received. On my first shift back, I was emailed by mistake by my CMW. She had meant to email my new manager. The 7 page document was hard to read. It outlined conversations she had had with members of staff. ***It had accusations that weren't true, in an attempt to undermine my new position on labour ward.*** *I sought support from a member of staff in the sluice who informed the band 7 and a formal complaint was made against my old manager. Head of Midwifery was informed and I began a formal complaint through the RCM and the local RCM representative for the unit was involved. To this day I feel this was all handled very hush hush, under the carpet and I was never informed of the outcome. I was asked what I wanted from the meeting. I said I would like an apology and an assurance that this would never happen to anyone else.* ***This never came and my manager rose to the rank of matron.*** *She has left the Trust now but I'm still left with dissatisfaction of how the complaint process was dealt with. I have all my documentation and the email if you* *would like this. Sorry for long message, I don't feel I've captured my experience through the same.*

Conclusion

Some accounts have been removed as it was not possible to anonymise them sufficiently to protect the identity of the individuals. Some accounts have had brief details removed to protect the anonymity of individuals.

These accounts from midwives provide first-hand accounts of how bullying is often being ignored in midwifery. Midwives also describe their experiences of racism and its impact on their health and well-being. Midwives have described their experiences of toxic cultures within their workplaces, with cliques, preferential treatment, unfounded allegations and poor working conditions leading to a negative impact on their health and well-being, including suicide attempts and midwives leaving their job and/or their profession. Those who do stay in their jobs and/or midwifery, often do so unwillingly for personal reasons. Many of the midwives who left midwifery did so reluctantly as it had previously been a long-held dream and they still believed passionately in the difference that high-quality midwifery care could make to the experiences and outcomes for women and babies.

Midwives' lives are being decimated and women and babies care is being negatively impacted. Long-term interventions that are resourced and sustained over months and years are needed to address this distressing and pervasive phenomenon.

Dr Patricia Gillen
Nurse, RGN, Midwife, RM, BSc Hons, PG Dip in ED, MSc, PhD, FHEA

References

Adams, A. (1992) *Bullying at Work: How to confront and overcome it London: Virago*

Bakker, A. B., & Demerouti, E. (2014). *Job demands-resources theory.* In P. Y. Chen & C. L.Cooper (Eds.), *Work and wellbeing* (pp. 37–64). Wiley Blackwell. **www.doi.org/10.1002/9781118539415.wbwell019**

Ball, L. Curtis, P. & Kirkham M. (2002) *Why do Midwives Leave?* London: RCM

Chatziioannidis I, Bascialla FG, Chatzivalsama P, Vouzas F, Mitsiakos G. *Prevalence, causes and mental health impact of workplace bullying in the Neonatal Intensive Care Unit environment.* BMJ Open. 2018 Feb 24;8(2):e018766. doi: 10.1136/bmjopen-2017-018766.

Einarsen, S. & Skogstad, A. (1996) Bullying at work: Epidemiological findings in public and private organizations *European Journal of Work and Organizational Psychology 5* (2) 185-201

Gillen, P. (2004) A concept analysis of bullying in midwifery *Evidence Based Midwifery 2* (2), 46-51

Gillen, P. (2008) *The nature and manifestations of bullying in midwifery* Belfast: Ulster University ISBN 13 978-1-85923-231-6

Gillen, P.A., Sinclair, M., Kernohan, W.G., Begley, C.M. and Luyben, A.G., 2017. Interventions for prevention of bullying in the workplace. *Cochrane database of systematic reviews,* (1).

Heinemann, P. (1972) Cited in: Olweus, D Sweden: IN Smith, P.K., Morita, T., Junger-Tas, J., Olweus, D., Catalano, R. and Slee, P. Eds The nature of School Bullying: a cross-national perspective, London: Routledge, 28-48

Keller, R., Allie, T. and Levine, R., 2019. An evaluation of the "BE NICE Champion" programme: A bullying intervention programme for registered nurses. *Journal of nursing management, 27*(4), pp.758-764.

Leyman, H (1996) The content and development of mobbing at work *European Journal of Work and Organizational Psychology* 5 (2), 164-184

Mulder, R., Bos, A.E., Pouwelse, M. and van Dam, K., 2017. Workplace mobbing: How the victim's coping behavior influences bystander responses. The Journal of social psychology, 157(1), pp.16-29.

Ng, K., Niven, K., & Notelaers, G. (2022). Does bystander behavior make a difference? How passive and active bystanders in the group moderate the effects of bullying exposure. Journal of Occupational Health Psychology, 27(1), 119 –135.**www.doi.org/10.1037/ocp0000296**

Niedl, K (1996) Mobbing and well-being: economic and personal development implications *European Journal of Work and Organizational Psychology* 5 (2), 239-249

Nielsen, M.B. and Einarsen, S.V., 2018. What we know, what we do not know, and what we should and could have known about workplace bullying: An overview of the literature and agenda for future research. Aggression and violent behavior, 42, pp.71-83.

Ockenden Maternity Review (2022) *Independent review of maternity services at the Shrewsbury and Telford Hospital NHS Trust. Final report: findings, conclusions and essential actions.* **www.ockendenmaternityreview.org.uk**

Paull, M., Omari, M. and Standen, P., 2012. When is a bystander not a bystander? A typology of the roles of bystanders in workplace bullying. Asia Pacific Journal of HumanbResources, 50(3), pp.351-366.

Royal College of Midwives (1996) *In place of Fear: Recognising and Confronting the problem of bullying in midwifery London*: RCM

Royal College of Midwives (2021) Making Maternity SErvices Safer: Human Facyors The Solution Series 3 London: RCM **www.rcm.org.uk/media/5182/the-solution-series-3-making-maternity-services-safer-human-factors.pdf**

Royal College of Nursing (2002) Working well? London: RCN

UNISON (1997) UNISON Members' experience of bullying at work London: UNISON Vartia, M (1996) The sources of bullying–psychological work environment and organizational climate European Journal of Work and Organizational Psychology 5 (2), 203-214

Walker, l.O. & Avant, K.C. (2005) *Strategies for Theory Construction in Nursing* 3rd ed Connecticut: Appleton Lange

Chapter 5:
The Role of the Unions in the Workplace

Whilst reading through all the experiences, the pain, suffering, disempowerment and destruction of each of the midwives, student midwives and maternity staff members telling their accounts becomes all too apparent. There is little mention of the systems that are in place actually making any positive or structural difference or protecting the staff. On the contrary, many accounts show that the systems that midwives expect to support them within the workplace and deal with the bullying and poor behaviours, end up being a futile "tick-box" exercise, which invariably ends up supporting the perpetrators. Nobody seems to have the wherewithal, courage or passion to tackle the poor culture effectively or much at all. There appears to be a "head in the sand approach".

This is a theme that occurs time and time again in these accounts. Alternatively, any changes are negligible and often work against the person who finds themselves in a more intolerable position than before. They may then both try to continue and learn to suffer in silence but find the intolerable behaviours continue (or intensify), and then they leave for another job or retire earlier than planned, risking long term financial disadvantage. Any of these solutions are viewed by unions and management as an acceptable/successful solution and the problem solved...but nothing has changed and poor culture continues unabated, where other midwives caught in the same trap lose any will to challenge the poor culture because they know it is futile, will make no difference and they increase the real risk of them becoming a target.

"It's safer to keep your head down or leave... *and we wonder why retention is so abysmal, maternity units have no staff and safety is compromised."*

Within the accounts, we quickly recognised that there was a recurrent theme of suboptimal union representation, or/and complicity with senior managers. Quite often a union representative wears at least two hats, for example, manager and union rep. This conflict of interest between roles was also described in the Morecambe

Bay report in 2015 (Kirkup, 2015). Accounts describe managers and unions being "friends and colleagues" who downplay or ignore the problem, leading to a lack of accountability, often blaming the complainant who may end up finding themselves with internal complaints against themselves, which are then pursued with gusto, often result in the midwife leaving. Again, the problem is deemed solved, by those in power.

This failure to tackle bullying at source, even when brave staff had given the unions the evidence with which to fight poor culture, can result in unions and Trusts investigating the bullying victim or whistle-blower rather than the perpetrator and brushing poor cultures and the evidence under the carpet. This approach further embeds poor culture. The Ockenden report (2022) found families and mothers who had witnessed poor working relationships which caused them additional stresses at one of the most vulnerable moments of their lives. Grievances are often downgraded to concerns and investigated internally, which puts the complainant at greater risk, reinforces poor behaviours and thereby, enables perpetrators to continue their reign of bullying, unabated and empowered.

Midwives who do leave because they feel they have no choice, generally have no exit interview and are not informed or supported to go to employment tribunals. Damaged and discarded midwives, some of whom will never recover, are not informed that they have an avenue of recourse through employment tribunals until it is too late - the time limit being 3 months minus 1 day precisely. After that, there is no recourse, but during this time limit, the midwife is often floundering, confused, suffering mental health issues, worried about finances and anxiety for the future and may understandably be unable to find the strength to continue. Midwives who do find a private solicitor to take their case on, face financial costs despite already paying substantial union fees for protection through their union solicitors.

The suboptimal management of bullying and culture does not just affect the midwife on the frontline. A separate, highly confidential and anonymised dossier which was shared only between the administrator of the #saynotobullyinginmidwifery group and the Chief Midwifery Officer of England in November 2021 included accounts from senior staff who described severe bullying and lack of support from within Trust management, and also University lecturers describe bullying within the academic world. The rot runs deep and unabated. This needs to change.

A union is described as a group of employees who join together to maintain and improve their conditions of employment (UNISON, nd.). Union representatives negotiate with members and employers on a number of issues, including (but not restricted to), pay, working conditions, supporting at grievances and disciplinary meetings. Unions have legal departments to help with legal and financial problems.

The Royal College of Midwives (RCM 2022) is both a trade union and a professional organisation with over 48,000 members, comprised of midwives, maternity support workers and student midwives in the United Kingdom. The RCM states that they are "the only professional organisation and trade union dedicated to serving midwifery and the whole midwifery team."As well as union representation, member benefits also include continuing professional development, education and training.

The Royal College of Nursing is both a trade union and a professional body, and has close to half a million nurses, midwives, nursing support workers and students as members. Membership offers education, an indemnity scheme, and workplace support. The RCN describes itself as "the Voice of Nursing." (RCN 2022)

Many midwives, particularly midwives who work outside the NHS system, are members of the RCN due to the RCN offering indemnity cover for antenatal and postnatal care, which is not offered by the RCM. Belonging to a union is relatively costly. At the time of publication, the RCM fees for an experienced, (qualified more than 1 year) midwife are £23.30 per month. Some midwives are joint members of the RCM and the RCN, which costs RCN members an additional £8.20 per month.

Other unions for health and public sector workers and academics in the UK include Unison (UK's largest trade union), Unite, UCU and the GMB. These unions are not professional organisations and are solely trade unions with trade union responsibilities.

The only union named in the accounts we received was the RCM.

In each chapter, we carefully anonymised the union names in the accounts as we felt they needed addressing in a separate section. Many accounts were submitted describing how midwives were in dire straits (or had left the profession) due to reasons of poor culture, bullying, excessive and unsafe workload, or no work-life balance, for example, but there was little evidence of the systems that are purported to be in place to protect them. Attempts to try and get support to resolve these problems appear futile or worse, counterproductive. Midwife after midwife was left unsupported and eventually as a last resort left the profession disempowered, disregarded and unvalued. We know that the current haemorrhage of the midwives from the NHS only adds to the lack of safety within our maternity units.

These instances and members' experiences are articulated in the following quotes, which have been anonymised earlier.

"The RCM holds major conflicts of interest – being a Union and Professional Body. EG Continuity of Care. The RCM may promote this as a professional body as best practice of care for a family, however as a Union, it is not necessarily safe and healthy for a midwife's mental health. Priority should be given to the Union side... protect staff and they will protect families in their care."

"I had spoken to a regional RCM rep from another area who was very helpful re looking at the Trust's bullying policy. I was advised to remain informal. A meeting was arranged with the Band 8 and Union Rep from RCM. I had contacted my regional RCM rep and asked if she could attend but was told I had to have one of the midwife reps. It is really incestuous as the Union Reps are all midwives working for the same trust and sometimes with the same colleagues that you have a grievance with so impartiality is difficult. Unfortunately the Regional Rep used to work for the Trust and is best friends with X who is close to Y so I was doomed from the start!"

"Just before I returned to work the RCM rep who had been supporting me went off with stress. I was told by the PMA that it was partially due to the time she spent supporting me as she was putting more work onto her colleagues and they did not like it. More blame and breach of confidence. She has just returned to work after 6 months off sick. Even though she was lovely, she was out of her depth."

"We had next to no support from our local RCM Rep."

"RCM as a body gave me minimal support to do what I needed to do, and virtually no hint of emotional support or concern when I ultimately moved on due to my actions working for their members on the shop floor. When I spelt out that ultimately I was being constructively dismissed, they ignored me and no support was offered. I now view them as complicit - or at least reluctant to take the sort of action that should have happened due to their very close and, in my opinion, biased relationships with the midwifery leaders across the UK. This makes them a union on paper only as far as I am concerned. I have found being a workplace rep to be extremely challenging and have often wondered how the RCM continues on when they provide such appalling counsel to their members and to the many reps who work so hard on the shop floor for little thanks."

"First I want to say a massive thank you for having these talks and being our advocate but my concern is where is our union in all this?"

"Whistle-blowers are not supported at any level, neither by their colleagues, nor management or union."

"What do you do when the bully has made herself almost untouchable? A midwife for several years AND has a role within the RCM. The repercussions for the person reporting this bullying (and their future in midwifery) feel immense, who would want to stand up against someone with a position within the RCM and have the perpetrator bad mouth you to their peers? I know of others who have been significantly bullied by midwives who are RCM reps. It seems becoming a rep, or higher within the RCM, is a way for bullies to protect themselves by ingratiating themselves with the very union who should protect midwives from bullying. I would also like to add that most RCM reps I've met are wonderful and caring midwives who are there to support us. I know they will be shocked and saddened by what I've written. It just feels like my bully protected herself from any accusations by being a rep, or gaining a higher position within the union, and this is also true of other people who've confided in me about the bullying they've had and have felt unable to report it because of the bully's position."

"I start with chronic bullying, union + trust management complicity, dishonest midwifery managers and poor and complicit union representation after whistle-blowing + raising public concerns."

"It's country wide. The RCM are as much use as a chocolate teapot."

"Therefore I decided I weren't prepared to tolerate this any longer and decided to get myself a union rep and instigate a meeting with the HoM. In the meeting she said I was the most challenging person she had met in a long time, as she had basically realised I wasn't cowering down to the coercive bullying tactics, or being forced into their nonsense corner, because I had checked out my right to apply for the role I was in before I had even applied. Therefore I knew what they were telling me to do was entirely unnecessary and wrong. They hadn't appreciated me thinking outside the usual midwifery "career path" box and wanted to make my life difficult. In the end I won my case as such, and I was eventually left alone."

"You may suggest that I would find solace and support from the RCM. When I tell you that I was a Rep where I worked, that I literally ruined my career because I knew I had to speak up and that in spite of everything, the RCM as a body gave me minimal support to do what I needed to do. When I spelt out that, ultimately I was being constructively dismissed, they ignored me and no support was offered."

"When these individuals are then able to further their careers and receive no repercussion even when their actions are questioned I am extremely concerned at the gravity of the repercussions of bullying when people also have the additional power to literally discipline you out of your job."

"I just wanted to tell you how high up the bullying and corruption goes and that it makes it very difficult to have any faith in the evolution of our services when those that lead do not hold the integrity and honesty that is required."

"Having been a qualified midwife for a fair few years I had naturally joined the RCM as this was promoted to us as early as university. I was subject to discrimination in the workplace, which spanned over years. It was subtle, corrosive and extremely damaging to my long term wellbeing. Having involved the RCM at the most convenient time, I expected more. I expected the union to rise as my advisor, advocate and professional protector. They did some lip service, then told me I should now be grateful for what the Trust were now doing for me. Irrelevant, in their opinion, that the law had been broken and their desire to support me had gone unfulfilled. They were noticeably inexperienced when it came to employment law. It was a devastating realisation, after all, these were midwives too. It's been a lengthy battle alone, one I will not give up on. I've banged down the doors of the union for a full refund, to no avail. In my opinion and from personal experience the RCM and trusts have conflict of interest. The RCM are poor advocates when educating members and the trust surrounding the equality act. It is evident there is poor leadership amongst midwifery managers and this is being filtered to the staff below. There is no doubt that this is contributing to the exodus of the remaining hard working, caring and dedicated midwives.

"Despite a huge volume of evidence, my bullying experiences at the hands of managers was downgraded by the union to a "dignity at work concern" which wasn't upheld. The bullying continued and I left the profession. I did approach

the union to reiterate that the bullying was the reason I was leaving and basically told "well you found out the hard way about trying to change things" and to just take it on the chin. I did not realise until later that I had a case for an employment tribunal. I have recently had my evidence (5 files) reviewed by an employment lawyer (at my own expense). My solicitor apologised for what I went through and acknowledged that I had had poor union representation. Nothing can be done but the closure is so important for me to now be able to move on."

"What people need to do now is to put in their own employment tribunal and find a solicitor as missing the date is the issue. They deliberately push you into the zone past 3 months minus 1 day, it just feels so corrupt."

"Despite paying RCM fees, when I was being bullied, I only found out all my options when I paid privately for solicitors advice myself. I feel stupid that I put my faith in the RCM. Most of my colleagues told me that the RCM were useless and that members fees were spent more on their public image, rather than helping members or improving working conditions."

In October 2022 the Report of the Independent Investigation into Maternity and Neonatal services in East Kent was published (Kirkup 2022). The report identified bullying, harassment and inappropriate behaviour within the Trust and maternity services had been prevalent over a prolonged period.

In 2014/15 the Head of Midwifery, along with HR did attempt to tackle the identified serious bullying problem within East Kent midwifery by conducting a review. The HoM and HR decided that some senior midwives who were repeatedly identified as central to the issues should be relocated or suspended pending further action. This led to a collective grievance with 49 signatories being submitted by the RCM, alleging failures of process in the review, although the RCM was already aware of the dysfunctional behaviours at the Trust.

As a result, the Trust withdrew support from the review process and from the Head of Midwifery. Consequently, the Head of Midwifery resigned from her post in August 2015. She requested advice from the RCM on whistleblowing about the culture of bullying and intimidation prevalent in the unit and was advised against disclosure in the interests of patient safety because of the risk this posed to her future career prospects. That former HoM told the Kirkup panel that she regretted going to the RCM for support with whistleblowing because the RCM advised them to resign and move on; if not, the RCM said that they would be unemployable in a senior position, and they should protect themselves. She told the Panel that it was really hard making the decision as she did not want to leave women vulnerable. However, she had been told by the RCM that whistleblowing was not in the public interest and she had to think of their career.

East Kent report identifies 4 areas for action. The NHS could be much better at:

- identifying poorly performing units
- giving care with compassion and kindness
- team-working with a common purpose
- responding to challenge with honesty

The Royal College of Midwives describe themselves as "the voice of midwifery." They are incredibly influential, not just in the UK but in global midwifery and maternity services. This Chapter highlights the voices of their members which it is vitally important for them to see recorded in black and white. The RCM need to reflect on the reason for their existence and integrity as a professional organisation and trade union. They state that they are 'dedicated to serving midwifery and the whole midwifery team' (RCM). The accounts included within this report do not reflect that perspective. It is time that the RCM do better! Time will tell if they are up to this challenge.

Amanda Burleigh
Midwife, RM, Nurse RGN, BSc Hons

References

Kirkup, B. (2015) *The Report of the Morecambe Bay Investigation*. The Stationary Office. London

Reading the signals: maternity and neonatal services in East Kent, the report of the independent investigation (print ready) (publishing.service.gov.uk) (Accessed 07/06/23)

Kirkup, B. (2022). *Reading the signals Maternity and neonatal services in East Kent-the Report of the Independent Investigation.* [online] Available at: **https://www.gov.uk/government/publications/maternity-and-neonatal-services-in-east-kent-reading-the-signals-report** (Accessed 24 Oct. 2022).

Ockenden, D. (30 March 2022) *Ockenden Review: Summary of findings, conclusions and essential actions, GOV.UK.* Available at: **www.gov.uk/government/publications/final-report-of-the-ockenden-review/ockenden-review-summary-of-findings-conclusions-and-essential-actions**
(Accessed 07/06/2023).

Royal College of Midwives (nd) About the RCM. Available at: **www.rcm.org.uk/about-us** (Accessed: November 7, 2022).

Royal College of Nursing (nd) Home: Royal College of Nursing Available at: **www.rcn.org.uk/** (Accessed: November 7, 2022).

What is a trade union?: What we do (2020) UNISON National. Available at: **www.unison.org.uk/about/what-we-do/about-trade-unions** (Accessed: November 15, 2022).

Chapter 6:
Reports and current strategies

For many midwives working in Great Britain and Northern Ireland, the Royal College of Midwives (RCM) is their union, while in the Republic of Ireland, it is the Irish Nurses and Midwives Organisation (INMO). In their research, Gillen et al., (2004) suggest that bullying is a complex phenomenon that crosses both personal and professional boundaries and thus these professional bodies have the capacity to speak out on behalf of their members.

One member of the '#saynotobullyinginmidwifery Facebook group' recalled the response from the RCM following their involvement:

"Head of Midwifery was informed, and I began a formal complaint through the RCM and the local RCM representative for the unit was involved. To this day I feel this was all handled very hush-hush, under the carpet and I was never informed of the outcome."

This midwife experienced bullying so severely, she considered taking her own life. Another midwife said,

"I know of others who have been significantly bullied by midwives who are RCM reps. It seems becoming a rep, or higher within the RCM, is a way for bullies to protect themselves by ingratiating themselves with the very Union who should protect midwives from bullying."

These quotes highlight how the input from the Workplace Union is not as supportive as expected.

'Following the findings of the Francis Inquiry into care at Mid Staffordshire Hospital (2013) which showed failure in the leadership of the hospital and a culture in which staff members reporting concerns about failure in care were discouraged from speaking out. The report also showed excess mortality of 400 to 1200 deaths, this inquiry also focused on maternity care. Findings such as this which recognized that failures and of poor working relationships between different groups of staff could be directly attributed to the deaths of eleven babies and one mother in Morecambe Bay Trust (2015), at the time the RCM issued a statement which sought to address the findings. More recently the Ockenden report found that a 'culture of fear' anxiety and bullying existed within maternity care at Shrewsbury and Telford Trust, resulting in staff fearing the consequences if they raised concerns.'

Staff bullying was a major factor in both investigations. The RCM and the RCOG (2014) published a toolkit which provided midwives and obstetricians with practical advice on actions they could take when experiencing bullying and undermining in the workplace. In 2015, the RCM launched the campaign 'Caring for You' (2016), which now exists in the form of an online hub where midwives can access a helpline and other supportive suggestions.

The RCM 'Caring for You' hub encourages midwives experiencing bullying to reach out to local representatives who will be able to provide support. In 2016, the RCM revisited the 2002 report, 'Why do Midwives Leave' with the survey 'Why midwives leave'. Nearly 20% cited bullying as a reason to leave, with 13% indicating bullying was initiated by a manager. This hub is only available to RCM members.

One member of the '#saynotobullyinginmidwifery Facebook group' recalled the response from the RCM following their involvement:

> *"I loved my job. I loved caring for women and sharing an incredible time of their lives with them. Understaffing and over-working I could cope with, but when you add in incredibly stressed-out colleagues and bullying supervisors then the good gets overshadowed. It's very sad."*
> *(#saynotobullyinginmidwifery Facebook group)*

The RCM commissioned the Work, Health, and Emotional Lives of Midwives (WHELM) study (2017) for midwives working in the United Kingdom (UK). In their investigation into the emotional well-being of midwives, the authors found that there were no 'quick fixes' to the problems causing burnout. However, they said the impact on midwives is deeply concerning, indicating that midwives' emotional well- being is now so compromised that two-thirds of those surveyed were considering leaving the profession. This study was to build on the 'Caring for You' campaign. One of the many findings of the WHELM study, included the most negative accounts from the participants, was bullying or undermining behaviour by managers, in front of women. Midwives also reported aggressive styles of management with lack of empathy and understanding. The report stated that, the RCM would use the robust data provided by their empirical study to press for change at the systems level while supporting the midwifery workforce to provide high quality compassionate care to women and families.

The UK has not been alone in this problem. In 2018, an online campaign was launched in Ireland to gather personal accounts from student midwives who have suffered bullying in Irish hospitals, in some cases severe enough to force them out of the profession. A survey of Trinity midwifery students from 2015 (Heaphy, Baker & Ring, 2015) showed almost 60 percent of respondents had experienced bullying while on placement in hospitals. The students reported how a rigid hierarchy, as well as staffing and retention pressures, have contributed to the bullying culture. Separate research conducted by the INMO between 2010 and 2014 found most respondents (51.9 per cent) reported experiencing bullying. One student admitted that after three years of hard study, sacrificing much of her personal life and simultaneously raising her three children, she decided to leave.

"became scared of the constant belittling of me as a person and as a student midwife. I dreaded seeing her coming into the ward."

In 2021, the RCOG and RCM recommitted to promoting a positive and safe working environment for all. Consideration, dignity, and respect for others were deemed as being essential to achieving this safe environment. In their statement, the RCM and the RCOG categorically condemned undermining and bullying behaviour under any circumstances. The initiative also saw the launch of the Workplace Behaviour Toolkit (2021), which has information for those who feel they have been bullied, those who witness bullying behaviour and those accused of being a bully.

Recognising that the issues of Birth Trauma are multifactorial, Patterson (2019), in her work on birth trauma, identified how bullying of midwives impacts on women's experience, with midwives feeling they must align themselves with obeying senior management and prioritising this over the needs of the women in their care. In describing the culture in maternity care as 'toxic and broken', despite calls from the RCM/RCOG for this extensive bullying culture to be addressed, negative behaviours by some midwives and managers have persisted. This culture impacts on women and their birthing experience, and Patterson strongly suggests that organisational issues such as, staffing, resources and the quality of the midwife-women relationship is essential for high quality care (Patterson, 2019).

On July 13th 2022, NHS England published a letter from the Chief Nursing Officer, Ruth May, which acknowledged that there is now a serious problem with retention of nurses and midwives in the NHS. While the letter seeks to address some of the issues with a five-point programme that sets out to improve career satisfaction thus improving retention, inclusion, and health and well-being, there is no mention of bullying despite the large percentage of midwives who identified it as a key reason for leaving the profession.

Whilst the RCM appears to be talking about acting on the reports/testimonials of workplace bullying the disturbing testimonials outlined in this report strongly indicate that there is a significant problem with the RCM's overall actions. In this report, both midwives and student midwives recall that, despite informing RCM representatives in their units of bullying on numerous occasions, they did not feel supported, with some feeling further ostracised for their actions. A wide gap remains between the organisational initiatives of their unions and what midwives experience in practice as union members. Whilst the RCM and the RCOG strongly encourage members to sign up for the 'Caring for You' and the 'Workplace Behaviour Toolkit', they remain optional. Individual accounts have stated that Heads of Midwifery have signed the caring for you charter in maternity units where bullying is known to be rife. It is essential that as well as signing the charter, mechanisms are in place to ensure that they are held accountable, as although a very important initiative, anybody can sign a charter and there needs to be evidence of good culture. This opting into such an important initiative may be part of the problem when sadly for those experiencing bullying the only option is to opt-out of their job and/or career.

Jeannine Webster, Midwife
RM, BSc in Midwifery, MSc in Health, and Social Care

References

Heaphy, E., Baker, S. & Ring, D. 2015 Report finds 60% of Midwifery Students Bullied on Placement, and Breach of Working Hours Agreement University Times. ie **www.universitytimes.ie/2015/06/report-finds-60-of-midwifery-students-buhttps://www.gov.uk/government/publications/final-report-of-the-ockenden-review/ockenden-review-summary-of-findings-conclusions-and-essential-actions** (Accessed 07/06/2023)

Hunter, B., Henley, J., Fenwick, J. et al (2018) Work, Health and Emotional Lives of midwives in the United Kingdom: The UK WHELM study **www.rcm.org.uk/media/2924/work-health-and-emotional-lives-of-midwives-in-the-united-kingdom-the-uk-whelm-study.pdf**

May, R. 2022 Letter, CNO, England **www.england.nhs.uk/publication/retaining-our-nursing-and-midwifery-colleagues**

O'Sullivan, S. (2002) Editorial Why do Midwives Leave **www.pubmed.ncbi.nlm.nih.gov/12154460**

Patterson J, Hollins Martin CJ, Karatzias T. Disempowered midwives and traumatised women: Exploring the parallel processes of care provider interaction that contribute to women developing Post Traumatic Stress Disorder (PTSD) post childbirth. Midwifery. 2019 Sep; 76:21-35. doi: 10.1016/j.midw.2019.05.010 . Epub 2019 May 25. PMID: 31154157

RCM & RCOG (nd) Workplace Behaviour Toolkit 2021 **www.rcog.org.uk/careers-and-training/starting-your-og-career/workforce/improving-workplace-behaviours/workplace-behaviour-toolkit** [last accessed 8/11/2022]

Royal College of Midwives (2016) Why Midwives Leavehttps: **www.britishjournalofmidwifery.com/content/birthwrite/reasons-why-midwives-leave** [last accessed 16/04/2023]

Royal College of Midwives (nd) **www.rcm.org.uk/caring-for-you-hub-home** [last accessed 8/11/2022]

Conclusion

The accounts in this report demonstrate how bullying in maternity services has managed to spread and permeate all areas of midwifery. The first chapter explores how even from the beginning of a midwife's career journey as a new student, it is common to experience or witness bullying and discriminatory behaviour. Then, if students do continue and successfully complete their training, often their working life as a newly qualified midwife can be blighted by a negative working environment and a bullying culture that seems to have been normalised in our maternity services workplaces. It should, however, also be acknowledged that these accounts also contained reports that pockets of kind and supportive midwives were encountered throughout midwifery training and life as a newly qualified midwife too.

When a newly qualified midwife consistently experiences a bullying culture in the workplace these accounts clearly reveal how quickly this can negatively impact upon how they feel in both their working and personal lives. Unhappy and toxic working environments can then reflect upon the type and quality of care which is provided for women and families using maternity services.

Cultural change during the formative years of midwifery training and the preceptorship of newly qualified midwives is therefore of paramount importance, not only to provide better, safer care for women and families but also to nurture and develop the careers of those who have invested themselves in this profession.

These students and newly qualified midwives are the future of midwifery and retaining them is not only cost effective and beneficial for the organisation, but ultimately provides better care for the women and families using the system.

The workload and continuity chapter provides accounts which display how heavy an impact bullying behaviour has on a midwife's working life, and how it can easily spill over into personal and family life. When midwives feel undervalued and are consistently not listened to by colleagues, managers and others about their concerns, it often leads them towards having to make tough choices about whether to stay in the career they have invested so much in, or to leave in order to protect their own mental and physical health and personal lives.

Biographies

#Saynotobullyinginmidwifery report team

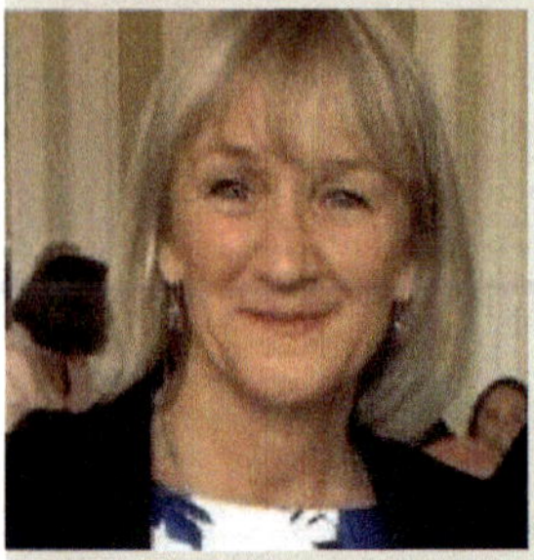

Amanda Burleigh

BSc Hons, Midwife RM, Nurse RGN

Ex Clinical Midwife. Author, Speaker, Midwifery Change Activist
Founder of Optimal Cord Clamping/waitforwhite (Facebook page and campaign).
Co-founder #Saynotobullyinginmidwifery (Facebook group + safe place to share about bullying).
Awards – Medical innovation Basics resuscitation trolley 2011 (team award)

- Midwife of the Year, Yorkshire Evening Post 2012
- Midwife of the Year, British Journal of Midwifery 2015

Amanda worked as a clinical midwife across a range of midwifery clinical settings (including New Zealand) for 29 years, before she left clinical midwifery in 2017 due to the effects of chronic bullying that she had endured since 2005 after identifying that the routine and recommended practice of immediate/early clamping of the umbilical cord had no evidence base to support safety of the intervention. On the contrary, the available research base shows immediate/early cord clamping causes harm particularly in premature and compromised infants. Amanda began campaigning for the implementation of evidence based practice around umbilical cord management but to this day has found there has been no accountability for the damage caused by decades of harmful, non-evidence based practice, which continues unabated globally and in the UK. In all reports investigating harm to babies, early clamping is not mentioned….it is the proverbial elephant in the room.

As a whistle blower and change activist, she suffered detriments to her mental and physical health, she witnessed such strong resistance to evidence based care and dishonesty amongst professionals that she no longer felt safe in her role as a midwife in this system, despite advocating for evidence based care, improving the safety of women, parents and babies.

Although Amanda is no longer employed as an NHS Midwife she remains a passionate registered midwife who continues to campaign globally for safe, evidence based umbilical cord management. Amanda is the founder of the global #waitforwhite campaign and now also campaigns against workplace bullying due to her own experiences.

Amanda was a Royal College of Midwives Board member from 2015-2018.

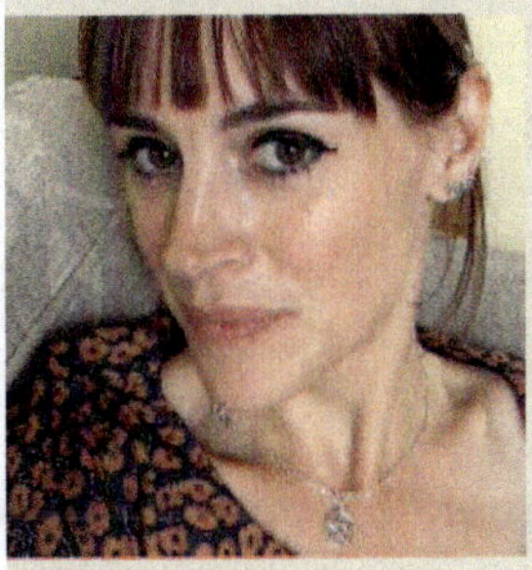

Jenny Wylam

BSc Hons (Midwifery), Midwife RM

On qualification, Jenny worked as a labour ward midwife until moving to focus on community midwifery in 2012. Later, this included leading a team of midwives working with the socially, culturally, and medically diverse population of London and, specifically within, one of the capital's most deprived boroughs.

Since 2017, Jenny has been working within her Trust's midwifery education team as a clinical practice facilitator. A huge part of this role is ensuring that student midwives undertaking their clinical placements at the Trust are supported to achieve the appropriate competence and confidence to successfully qualify at the end of their training.

Alongside this role, Jenny works as a clinical teacher within the midwifery department of a London university. As well as simulation-based teaching and assessment of fundamental and life-saving midwifery skills and theory, within her role, she also provides pastoral support and guidance to many of the students undertaking their midwifery studies there.

Jenny first joined the #saynotobullyinginmidwifery group in 2020 having witnessed, personally experienced, stood up to, and resolved incidences of bullying over the years. She is passionate in believing that the only way maternity services can be truly safe for women and babies is if they prioritise the care and support of midwives as PEOPLE, and value and nurture this most precious asset.

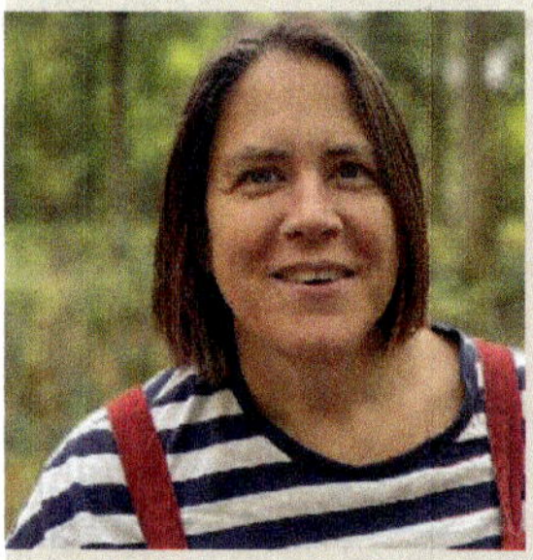

Becky Millar

BSc Hons Nursing (adult). BSc Hons Midwifery
MSc Advanced Practice Student

Becky has worked predominantly within the Midwife Led setting and Community Midwifery, in-cluding within a Team Caseloading model. She is passionate about supporting informed choice for place of birth and decision making. Becky joined the Association of Radical Midwives as a student and has served two terms on the steering group. As a Supervisor of Midwives and Professional Midwifery Advocate Becky has supported both families and staff with complex care planning and incident investigations.

Since 2019 Becky has been the Better Births Project Midwife responsible for implementation of Midwifery Continuity of Carer and other Maternity Transformation Program workstreams to change practice and develop improvements.

Witnessing, experiencing, and supporting friends and colleagues with issues within the workplace led Becky to join the 'say no to bullying in midwifery' Facebook group. She was disturbed by the reports and experiences of midwives, the quantity and extent of which have shown that toxic culture and bullying in midwifery is endemic and must be addressed in order to protect individuals and our maternity service.

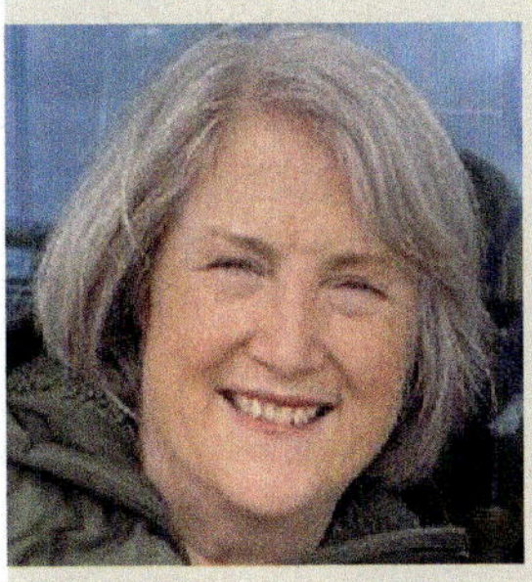

Dr Patricia Gillen

PhD, MSC, PGDipE, BSC (Hons), Midwife RM, Nurse RN, FHEA

Dr Patricia Gillen (PhD) is a registered nurse and midwife who has worked across a range of clinical settings, been a delivery suite sister and managed a rural maternity unit. Patricia has worked in academia and in a joint post between the Southern Health and Social Care Trust as Head of Research and Development for Nurses, Midwives and AHPs and as a Reader in the School of Nursing, Ulster University. She has just completed 8 years as a UK representative for the European Midwives Association.

Patricia has led on research into women and healthcare providers' experiences of home birth. She has led and contributed to a UK wide study which explored health and social care workers self-report on well-being and coping during COVID-19.

Patricia's explored the nature and manifestations of bullying in midwifery for her PhD and led on a Cochrane Review of the Effectiveness of Interventions to Prevent Bullying in the Workplace (2017).

Patricia previously served two terms as the elected Chair of the RCM Board (2011-2015) and on the NMC Midwifery Committee (2014-2017). Patricia has personally experienced bullying as a nurse, midwife and academic, in both practice and university settings. These experiences have in part led to her leaving jobs and have impacted on her career progression.

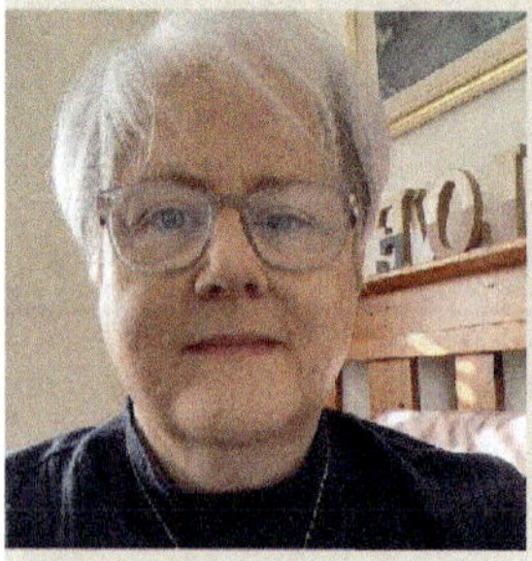

Jeannine Webster

BSc in Midwifery, MSc in Health and Social Care, Midwife (with a disability)

Founder and PRO Midwives Association of Ireland. Women's Choice and Mental Health Advocate. Proponent for improvements in maternity care and recognition of the role midwives can/do play in these improvements. Espouser for recognition of bullying in midwifery, and in particular student midwives. Member of REFOCUS committee in the Irish College of Psychiatrists.

Jeannine is currently involved with Women's Aid Maternity Project, and National Obstetric Guideline Committee updating the guidance on screening for Domestic Violence in Pregnancy. Jeannine is also currently on the HSE guideline committee for Domestic Violence in pregnancy.

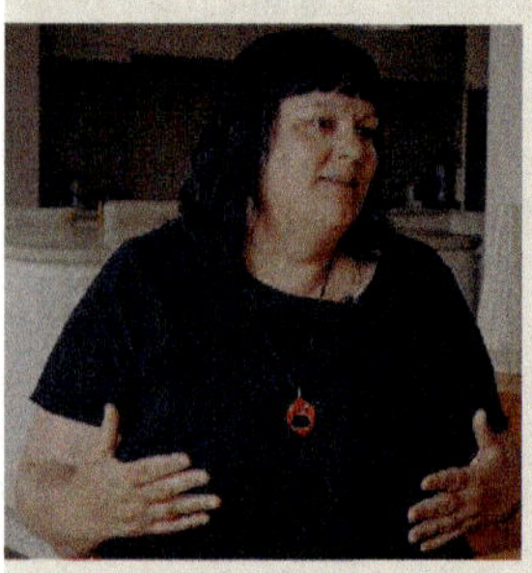

Karen McEwen

BSc Midwifery, MSc Clinical Research Methods, Midwife RM

After qualifying as a midwife in 2007, Karen's career has focussed on intrapartum care for women in inner city delivery suites, alongside and stand-alone birth centres, having a particular interest in helping women and families achieve better and more positive birth experiences, whether that be in the hospital or the community. During this time, she helped to found and develop a homebirth team in West Yorkshire, which also supported women choosing to birth outside of hospital guidelines.

She has also invested time developing waterbirth teaching packages and guidelines to support midwife teams to become confident in offering water and waterbirth to women during labour, as well as being involved in implementing delayed cord clamping guidelines.

She became a member of the Facebook group #saynotobullyinginmidwifery after both witnessing and experiencing a culture of bullying throughout her career, and became involved in developing this report in the hope of playing a part in tackling this problem in midwifery in the future.

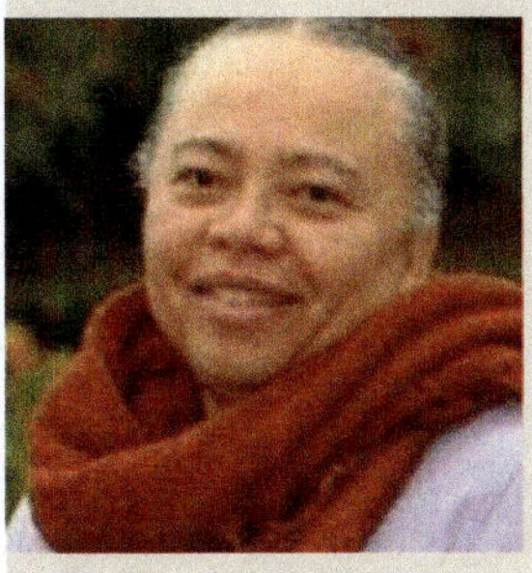

Elsie Gayle

Honorary Fellow, University of Wolverhampton

Elsie Gayle is a midwife in private practice in the United Kingdom; having significant national and international experience.

She focusses on delivering 'culturally safe' maternity care; which simply helps any woman to choose services to meet their needs and values.

The model is dedicated to ameliorate the historical roots of inequalities in service provision, obstetric violence and the poor outcomes for disadvantaged mothers and babies, especially those of African descent.

She initiated 'Midwifery Conversations' to support a wide network of clinicians, students and interested others in the birth world. It facilitates learning, updating clinical and regulatory practices.

In 2016 she presented maternal and baby mortality/morbidity findings to the United Nations (UN) Committee for Elimination of Racial Discrimination (CERD) in Geneva, alongside the Global African Congressuk (GACuk) where she now occupies the position of Honorable Elder and Secretary of that Committee.

Receiving Honorary Fellowship of the University of Wolverhampton in 2017, recognised Elsie's contribution, passion and commitment for midwifery, women's rights in childbirth and mental health services within the Black community.

In 2019 Iolanthe 'Jean Davies' Award allowed Elsie to host the first UK, international 'Reproductive Sankofa

Conference' to begin the in-depth work of repairing the poor maternity care issues for women of African descent.

She is Co-Secretariat to the All Party Parliamentary Group on Black Maternal Health.

Currently Elsie is engaged with the Inauguration of The United Nations Permanent Forum for People of African Descent, working alongside the Education and Outreach Sub-Committee

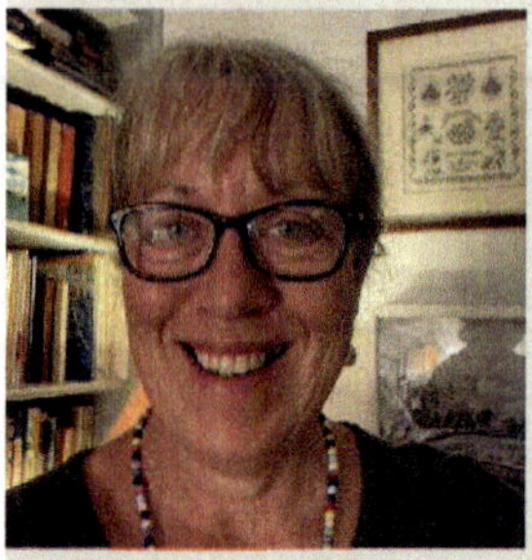

Deborah Hughes
BA(Hons) SRN RM MA PGDE

Co-ordinator of The Midwives Haven, Association of Radical Midwives

Deborah qualified as a nurse in 1980 and as a midwife in 1982. She practised midwifery for 40 years to 2022, as a hospital and community midwife, an independent midwife, a midwifery lecturer, a manager in a Sure Start Project, in two birth centres, a community midwifery manager, and a research midwife. She has been a RCM Steward, a Supervisor of Midwives, a Hypnobirthing teacher, and is a qualified homeopath. She has written extensively on midwifery and related topics in academic and professional journals, and is the author of a book on gestational diabetes and the co-author of another on why birth centres fail.

She co-founded The Midwives Haven **www.midwifery.org.uk/midwives-haven** with Angie Barrett in 2017 after they became concerned about the devastating and counter-productive consequences for midwives and the profession of the punitive and adversarial professional regulation of midwifery and fitness to practise processes. Realising that many NMC referrals originate in bullying cultures, she joined #Saynotobullyinginmidwifery. She also helped organise and spoke at the national conference on bullying in midwifery which took place in Bradford in 2012. Some of her research work also focussed on the culture of midwifery.

Deborah is particularly concerned at the bullying of newly qualified midwives and the impact of this on future practice, and the systematic bullying of independent midwives by professional institutions.

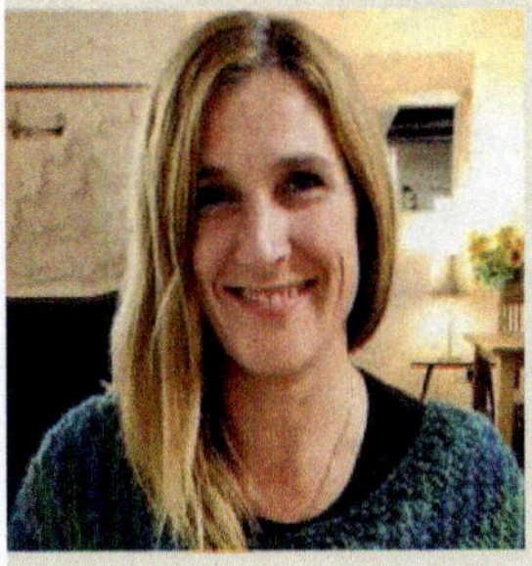

Andrea Lawrie
B Midwifery, PG Cert LTA, FHEA, Midwife RM

Andrea is a Registered Midwife and Registered Midwifery Teacher who, throughout her career, has worked clinically across a diverse range of hospital and community settings, including managing a successful midwife-led birth unit. As a student, Andrea was elected as a representative of the Royal College of Midwives (RCM) Student Midwife Forum where she supported several students who experienced bullying and undermining behaviours during their clinical placements. Once qualified, Andrea went on to become a Workplace Behaviour Champion, where she continued to advocate for students and staff alike. As part of a team, Andrea worked on a collaboration project with the RCM and Royal College of Obstetrician & Gynaecologists creating an online Workplace Behaviour Toolkit which aimed to raise awareness of bullying and undermining behaviours and encouraged staff and students to report and seek support. Andrea's passion for education and desire to make a difference to the experience and retention of student midwives, led to her current career in midwifery education.

Acknowledgements

We are very grateful to a number of people who have supported us with the contributions, development, editing, proof reading and publication of this report.

These include (in alphabetical order) but are not limited to:

ARM Steering Group, Lady A., Angie Barrett (Co-ordinator Midwives Haven, Association of Radical Midwives), Dr Jane Clossick, Dany Griffiths (co-founder #saynotobullyinginmidwifery) Jules Haigh (Lead Digital Midwife, RIP), Kay King (Movement Director at White Ribbon Alliance UK), Professor Mavis Kirkham, Maddie McMahon (Doula and Breastfeeding counsellor), Dr Jo Murphy-Lawless, (University College Galway), Cheryl Samuels (Midwifery Lecturer), Professor Mary Steen, TIMBET (The Independent Midwifery, Birth & Education Trust), Dr Sara Wickham.

And of course to all the members of the #saynotobullyinginmidwifery group.

Thank you, these are your voices

Printed in Great Britain
by Amazon

31678446R00089